SECOND OPINIONS IN
INTERNAL MEDICINE

AF085626

SECOND OPINIONS IN INTERNAL MEDICINE

by

Gerald Sandler
Consultant Physician
Barnsley District General Hospital
Barnsley, UK

and

John Fry
General Practitioner, Beckenham, Kent, UK

with

Wesley Fabb
General Practitioner, Rosanna, Victoria, Australia and
Secretary of WONCA

and

Martin Godfrey
Group Medical Editor, Haymarket Publications
General Practitioner, Beckenham, Kent, UK

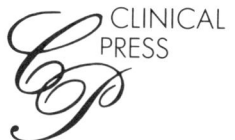

© Clinical Press Limited 1990

All rights reserved. No part of this publication may be reproduced, stored in a retrieval system, or transmitted in any form or by any means, electronic, mechanical, photocopying, recording or otherwise, without the prior permission of the Copyright Owner.

Published by Clinical Press Limited,
Redland Green Farm, Redland Green, Redland, Bristol, BS6 6HF

British Library Cataloguing in Publication Data
Second opinions in internal medicine. (Clinical handbooks)
   1. Patients. Referral by General Practitioners
   I. Sandler, Gerald, *1928–*   II. Fry, John, *1922–*
616

ISBN: 1-85457-019-6

Lasertypeset by Martin Lister Publishing Services, Carnforth, Lancs

Printed in the UK by Butler & Tanner Limited, Frome and London

Contents

	Preface	vii
1.	Jaundice	1
2.	Resistant high blood pressure	13
3.	Breathlessness	25
4.	Persistent dyspepsia	35
5.	Mrs 'Never Well'	47
6.	Headaches	57
7.	Swollen legs	67
8.	Multiple joint pains	77
9.	Chest pain	89
10.	Funny turns	101
11.	Dizziness	115
12.	Back pain	125
	Index	137

Preface

No doctor can work alone. There is always need to consult with colleagues to ensure good patient care. As a generalist, the family doctor develops his own skills and methods for the common problems he manages well, but occasionally there is need for a "second opinion" in consultation with a specialist colleague and to call on his, or her, special experience. Following such a consultation, the patient returns to the long-term care of the family doctor.

Little attention has been paid to the intricacies of the process of second opinions. There have been studies on the rates of referrals by British general practitioners to specialists, and wide ranges of differences have been found, but none has explored: why a referral is made, and how and to whom? What communications? What outcomes and benefits?

We have approached the subject in a novel but logical manner. The family doctor gives a case history of each of 12 common clinical medical problems from his practice, which he refers to his specialist internist colleague who analyses and assesses the problem and reports back.

We follow the same format for each problem –

- clinical presentation and assessment by the family doctor giving reasons for the referral
- the communication by letter
- the specialist's assessment and evaluation of the problem
- his report to the family doctor
- the outcome of the case

PREFACE

In addition, we interrupt the text by posing questions to the reader, by noting lessons learnt by both family doctor and specialist and lists of suitable topics for small group discussions.

We dedicate our book to family medicine trainees and their teachers, highlighting this important interface between primary and secondary medical care, but we hope that teachers of medical students will use it in outpatient departments in discussing referrals from family doctors.

We have worked as a team with JF providing cases from his practice, and GS responding, and with MG and WEF commenting and advising.

Gerald Sandler
John Fry
Wesley Fabb
Martin Godfrey

1 Jaundice

DENIS M (AGE 51)

A light vehicle driver delivering local goods for a large national company and acting as a part-time mini-cab driver.

Normally very fit and, apart from an appendictomy in his teens, he has not been seen very often.

He has been unwell for 3 days with 'flu'. Now feeling better but has noted 'dark urine'. Faeces are normal in colour. No abdominal discomfort.

He denies any nausea or anorexia. He has not been overseas over the past year, he has not had any injections or blood products. He does not eat out.

He drinks beer only at week-ends, about 4 pints (8 units) on Saturday and Sunday. Non-smoker.

The only unusual event in the past 2 weeks was that he was summoned for a medical check-up at work. There he was told he had 'high blood pressure' and given atenolol 100 mg to be taken daily (there has been no communication from the company doctor yet).

Examination

Very healthy appearance
Not overweight

Conjunctivae yellow tinged
No jaundice apparent in skin
Nil abnormal in abdomen
BP 140/68 CVS normal
Rectal examination normal, faeces on finger stall brown in colour
Urine dark with bile pigment

- What are the possible diagnoses?
- What life-style habits should be considered further?
- What views on the work check-up?

MANAGEMENT

Advised to rest and stay away from work. To stop antenolol. No new medication given. Liver function tests ordered. Significant findings were:

Alkaline phosphatase	440 U/l (normal 20–110)
Bilirubin	113/µmol/1 (3–21)
Alanine aminotransferase	507 IU/l (11–55)

- What other advice would you give?
- What other questions/investigations?

The GP's assessment

Dennis M is a fit man with recent jaundice and with no previous history of gastrointestinal disorders.

He is a light drinker and does not indulge in drug taking. He has not been overseas. Rest of his family and colleagues at work are all well.

He has been on atenolol for 2 weeks. His BP is normal.

Is this an infective hepatitis, a medication-jaundice or what else?

JAUNDICE

> - What do you say to Mr M?
> - Would you refer at this stage or do more yourself?

REFERRAL TO CONSULTANT

Dear Gerald,

Dennis M (51)
A 'jaundice' for you to sort out!
Mr M came to see me a week ago with a 3-day history of general malaise and fever for 2 days.

When I first saw him his conjunctivae were yellow and urine dark with bile pigment, faeces brown.

Now a week later he is feeling better, urine is normal in colour but conjunctivae still lemon-tinted.

I can find no causes for his jaundice in his life-style, i.e. light drinker, non-smoker, no drug history, sexually has never been homosexual or promiscuous, not been overseas recently.

The only possible cause apart from an infective hepatitis is that he was given atenolol 100 mg daily for 2 weeks (by his work doctor) for 'high blood pressure'. I have never found a raised BP – today it is 136/80 (he has been off atenolol for a week). Liver function tests (a week ago) showed:

bilirubin	440 µ/l	(3-21)
alkaline phosphatase	113 µmol/l	(20-110)
ALT	507 IU/l	(11-55)

I have not yet had results of tests for Hepatitis B.

Although he seems to be recovering naturally I am seeking your help for two reasons:
1. *For your views on the likely diagnosis and management.*
2. *Because he is rather angry at the work doctor putting him on atenolol with no good evidence that he has hypertension and without letting us know.*

Yours,

John

> • What is your opinion of this referral letter?

CONSULTANT ASSESSMENT

The clinical problem is acute jaundice in a previously fit patient who had also been found recently to be hypertensive and had started atenolol treatment.

There are two problems to be considered in this patient: (a) recent onset of jaundice; (b) asymptomatic hypertension.

Jaundice

The main causes of jaundice are:

- hepatitis – acute and chronic
- gallstones
- carcinoma of pancreas
- hepatotoxic drugs
- haemolytic anaemia – congenital and acquired

The first decision, therefore, to be made in a jaundiced patient is the type of jaundice which is present and the clinical features which may help are shown in Table 1.1

Table 1.1 Clinical features of jaundice

	Haemolytic	Hepatocellular	Obstructive
Jaundice	Mild	Mild–moderate	Severe
Symptoms	Nil (except in crisis)	Anorexia Malaise Distaste for smoking	Itching
Urine	Dark	Normal or dark	Dark
Stools	Dark	Normal or pale	Pale

JAUNDICE

Analysis of the GPs findings in relation to the jaundice

History

The flu-like illness which preceded the onset of the jaundice is suggestive of the prodromal phase of infective hepatitis even though he denies anorexia and nausea.

The absence of any recent injections or blood transfusion makes infection with hepatitis B unlikely: if he does have hepatitis this would favour hepatitis A infection or possibly non-A non-B.

The moderate weekly intake of beer makes alcoholic cirrhosis very unlikely.

The dark urine indicates excessive urinary urobilinogen excretion as a result of some biliary obstruction, but the normal colour of the stools shows that the degree of the obstruction is not very severe.

He has recently started atenolol: beta-blockers have not so far been known to cause jaundice. He has not taken any other potentially hepatotoxic drugs such as:

Psychotropic	• monoamine oxidase inhibitors
	• tricyclic anti-depressants
	• phenothiazines
	• benzodiazepines
Anti-inflammatory	• NSAIDs
	• penicillamine
	• gold
Antihypertensive	• methyl-dopa
	• hydrallazine
Antidiabetic	• chlorpropamide
Anticonvulsant	• phenytoin
Antibiotic	• sulphonamides
	• nitrofurantoin
	• isoniazid

Examination findings

The jaundice is evident in the conjunctivae: the absence of scratch marks excludes any significant obstruction. There is no abdominal abnormality to suggest:

cirrhosis	• enlarged liver
	• enlarged spleen
	• dilated veins
	• ascites
chronic active hepatitis	• enlarged liver
ca pancreas	• epigastric mass
	• distended gallbladder
gallstones	• Murphy's sign
liver metastases	• enlarged nodular liver

The normal colour of the stool on rectal examination suggests there is no serious obstructive jaundice.

GPs investigations

Liver function tests: the increased billirubin confirms the jaundice though there is no indication of whether it is the pre-hepatic (indirect) bilirubin which is increased – as in haemolytic jaundice – or the post-hepatic (direct) bilirubin – indicative of intra- or extrahepatic obstruction.

The normal alkaline phosphatase excludes significant obstruction (cholestasis).

The raised ALT indicates hepatocellular damage.

These results are consistent with hepatocellular jaundice which could result from either acute or chronic hepatitis, including cirrhosis.

Analysis of the GPs findings in relation to the hypertension

The important decisions to make in regard to Mr M's hypertension – as indeed with any patient's hypertension – are:

- whether it is primary (essential) or secondary
- whether there is target or organ damage
- whether it requires any treatment

Primary or secondary hypertension?

There is no mention of whether Mr M comes from a hypertensive family. Since 90–95% of all hypertensive patients in practice have essential hypertension and this is frequently associated with a positive family history this information should be sought. If the hypertension is secondary, the commonest cause is renal disease; there is no past history of kidney disease in Mr M or current urinary symptoms, which make a diagnosis of hypertension secondary to renal disease unlikely. Examination has not shown any evidence of Cushing's disease but there is no mention of delayed or absent femoral pulses associated with scapular pulsation which might suggest coarction of the aorta.

Target organ damage

The main target organs are heart, brain and kidneys. Involvement of any of these organs would reinforce the need for effective blood pressure control. There is no angina or breathlessness to suggest cardiac involvement, no previous stroke and, as mentioned above, no past history of kidney disease or current urinary symptoms to implicate the kidneys.

Although the GP's examination has shown a normal blood pressure there is a history of a raised blood pressure at work, and since hypertension is a frequent accompaniment of renal disease it would be advisable to investigate this further. The normal abdominal examination has excluded polycystic disease, which is an important, though rare, cause of secondary hypertension. It is not clear whether a renal artery murmur was sought as this abdominal sign may sometimes be overlooked in a hypertensive patient.

Does Mr M require treatment for hypertension?

There are some clear indications for treating hypertension:

- malignant hypertension
- target organ damage
- the level of the blood pressure
- systolic – over 160 mmHg
- diastolic – over 90 mmHg

When the blood pressure is only mildly elevated then the factors which should be taken into consideration before deciding whether to start treatment are:

- male patient, especially if young
- bad family history of hypertension, coronary or cerebrovascular disease
- other adverse risk factors
- cigarette smoking
- high blood cholesterol
- diabetes

Dr Fry does not know what level of blood pressure was found when Mr M was checked at work but his own blood pressure reading was normal. It is obvious that several further readings need to be taken over the course of the next few weeks before the question of treatment can be sensibly considered.

The family history is not mentioned in Dr Fry's letter and will therefore have to be sought.

JAUNDICE

Mr M does not smoke. His blood cholesterol level will need checking as will the blood sugar to make sure he is not a latent diabetic.

- From this assessment what is the likely cause?
- Would you treat his BP?

CONSULTANT'S LETTER TO THE GP

Dear John,
Thank you for referring this patient for assessment primarily of his jaundice, but also with a secondary problem of asymptomatic hypertension found during a routine medical check at work which so far you have been unable to confirm.

I have gone over the history with him and examined him carefully but can add little in the way of positive findings to your own assessment. There were no past history, symptoms or signs to suggest chronic liver disease such as cirrhosis or chronic active hepatitis, and nothing to indicate malignancy due to carcinoma of the pancreas or hepatic metastases. With regard to your question about possible hepatotoxic effects of atenolol, to the best of my knowledge there are no reports of this association.

I think therefore that the most likely diagnosis is infective hepatitis. This is supported by the prodromal symptoms and the results of the liver function tests which indicate hepatocellular damage and no significant cholestatic problem.

I am arranging for viral studies for hepatitis A, B and non-A non-B and will let you have the result when it is to hand. I do not think it will significantly affect management except in so far as a positive hepatitis B result will indicate the need for long-term supervision for the development of chronic active hepatitis, which occurs in 3–5% of patients.

There is little to be done in the way of active treatment for acute hepatitis beyond avoiding alcohol. Most cases will resolve spontaneously within a few weeks at the most: if Mr M does not settle satisfactorily within this time he will require further investigation including a liver biopsy.

Now to turn to the problem of the hypertension. There is no family history of hypertension to suggest a liability to essential hypertension, neither is there a family history of premature vascular disease. There is no clinical evidence of past or present renal disease to suggest secondary hypertension and I could not hear a renal murmur on abdominal examination to indicate renal artery stenosis. With respect to the rarer causes of hypertension, there are no symptoms of phaeochromocytoma (paroxysmal headache, sweating, palpitations, tremor), nor is there any weakness and polyuria to suggest primary or secondary hyperaldosteronism with hypokalaemia, and the femoral pulses were normal excluding coarctation. Like you, I found his blood pressure normal at 135/75 but it would obviously be advisable to obtain some more readings over the next few weeks. If the pressure remains normal I do not think we need to take any further action, but if it rises again, it is desirable to assess his target organs – chest X-ray to assess heart size, ECG for left ventricular hypertrophy and blood urea and serum creatinine levels for renal involvement. Additional risk factors, such as cholesterol and blood sugar, should also be measured before coming to any decision about treatment, especially if the hypertension is only mild.

I have not arranged another routine appointment for him but I would be glad to see him again any time if you feel it would be helpful.

Yours,

Gerald

- What is your opinion of this letter?

JAUNDICE

OUTCOME

Within 3 weeks the jaundice had cleared. The blood test report was:

Bilirubin	12 μmol/l (3–21)
Alk. Phosphatase	82 IU/l (20–110)
ALT	21 IU/l (11–55)

Serology report was:

Hepatitis B antigen	Negative
Hepatitis A IgM antibody	Negative
Hepatitis A IgG antibody	Positive

Therefore, Dennis M had had hepatitis A infection.

PRACTICAL ISSUES

- Most cases of jaundice can be managed, at least initially by the GP, providing that he has access to a good pathology service.
- Although hepatitis A is termed 'infective' or 'epidemic' in an urban community it is usually sporadic and the causal site rarely defined.
- Dennis M must be given general advice on his future in relation to his recent hepatitis.
- What advice?

SUBJECTS FOR GROUP DISCUSSION

- Relations between GP and occupational physicians.
- Criteria for starting treatment with antihypertensives.
- Public health measures in hepatitis infections.

2 Resistant High Blood Pressure

MRS E (AGED 55)

Well known in the practice for over 30 years. Married with two children.

During her pregnancies, over 20 years ago, her blood pressure was raised and has persisted high. Since 1965 her blood pressure has ranged from 220/120 to 180/105.

She is overweight, a non-smoker and non-drinker. There is a happy stable background. Her parents are still alive in their late 70s.

Mrs E is a busy extrovert in local voluntary work. She never complains and is always 'fine'.

Investigations

Chest X-ray: no cardiac enlargement, clear lung fields
ECG: normal
Urine: no protein or sugar

MANAGEMENT

Management has consisted of efforts to reduce her weight – without success (her parents and her brother are all 'large').

As she has been free of symptoms and with no signs of hypertensive disease, no great efforts were made to control her raised blood pressure with drugs.

However, in view of current medical opinion it was decided that an attempt should be made to reduce her blood pressure.

Over the past 5 years she has been prescribed:

bendrofluazide	5 mg daily
propranolol	up to 240 mg daily
nifedipine	up to 60 mg daily

In spite of this medication her blood pressure remains little altered at 200/110 to 170/105

> - Would you continue Mrs E's present treatment and modest blood pressure control or do you think her management should be altered – if so, why?

My anxiety is that Mrs E has had a moderately high blood pressure for over 20 years and I have been unable to control it. She is at risk of a stroke. I believe it is necessary to seek a second opinion.

> - Why refer for a second opinion – after all this time?

REFERRAL LETTER

Dear Gerald,

Mrs Joan E
I seek your advice with Mrs E whom I have known for many years.

RESISTANT HIGH BLOOD PRESSURE

The problem is her persistent high blood pressure in spite of my efforts to control it with bendrofluazide 5 mg, propranolol up to 240 mg and nifedipine up to 60 mg daily. It is 210/110 today.

She is a happy uncomplaining person with no apparent problems. She is overweight but has been unable to reduce it. There are no abnormal signs in heart or fundi and urinalysis is normal. She does not smoke or drink alcohol. There is no adverse family history.

My reasons for referral to you are:
- *my failure to control her high blood pressure*
- *my hope that you may be able to tell me why I have failed*
- *my expectation that you will suggest some more effective management*
- *my request that you explain the situation to Mrs E and give her your views on her prognosis.*

Yours,

John

- Do you think that this is a good referral letter and that all the relevant points have been made to the consultant? Have the right questions been asked?

CONSULTANT'S ASSESSMENT

Clinical significance of high blood pressure

Epidemiological data has shown quite clearly that persistently raised blood pressure, even of a mild degree, is associated with increased risk of stroke, left ventricular failure, renal failure and accelerated atherosclerosis. Furthermore controlled clinical trials have shown that treatment of mild to moderate hypertension does significantly reduce the likelihood of stroke but not of heart attacks, and there is no overall reduction in mortality.

However, deciding the potential risk of stroke or other vascular event in individual patients like Mrs E is much more difficult and must be based on a thorough clinical assessment of Mrs E with particular reference to:

- the presence of *other vascular risk factors* which increase the need for effective treatment because they enhance the development of atheroma (bad family history, smoking, hyperlipidaemia, diabetes, obesity, oestrogens for menopausal symptoms).
- the presence of *target organ damage* (heart, brain, kidneys) which also increase the need for more satisfactory blood pressure control.

Mrs E's case
Associated risk factors

We know that Mrs E has a good family history, is a non-smoker and probably not a diabetic (no glycosuria). She is, however, obese and we do not know her blood cholesterol level – this should be checked.

Target organ damage

Initial assessment by John Fry has shown no clinical evidence of target organ damage and the normal heart X-ray and ECG excludes cardiac involvement. The absence of urinary protein, however, does not exclude renal damage and her blood urea and creatinine levels should be checked.

The problems of resistant hypertension

There are three important considerations:

- compliance
- is the hypertension secondary
- are there any 'drug-neutralizing' factors

Compliance

Before accepting that a hypertensive patient is resistant to treatment it is necessary to ensure that the patient is taking all the drugs prescribed and that the drugs are given in adequate dose. With beta-blockers this is easy since the patient's resting pulse rate should be 60/min or less and the exercise rate <120/min. With diuretics there should be a fall in body weight and a fall in serum potassium level. Other hypotensive drugs are difficult to assess on a clinical basis.

Is the hypertension secondary?

Between 90 and 95% of hypertensive patients are 'essential' and the cause is unknown. However, there is an underlying primary cause in the remainder which may lead to resistance to treatment and so a search should be made for:

renal disease	• parenchymatous
	• renal artery stenosis
endocrine disorders	• phaeochromocytoma
	• Conn's syndrome
	• Cushing's syndrome
coarction of the aorta	

The importance of this search is underlined by the fact that most of these conditions are surgically remediable.

Are there are other factors interfering with treatment response?

- Is there excessive fluid retention (leg oedema and weight gain)?
- Is the patient taking too much salt?

- Is the patient taking other drugs – sympathomimetics, steroids, oestrogens, non-steroidal anti-inflammatory drugs. tricyclic antidepressants?

Mrs E's case

The possibility of an underlying primary cause for her hypertension is unlikely after 20 years with no symptoms and a negative clinical examination, and special tests for endocrine disorders are not indicated. An IVP may, however, be useful as chronic kidney disease can be asymptomatic for a long time. If the IVP is normal and Mrs E has been taking her drugs conscientiously and she is on no other treatment which might interfere with the action of these drugs then the possible factors which may be causing drug resistance are:

- the obesity
- inadequacy of the dose of propranolol – this should be assessed on resting and exercise pulse rate as described.
- the drugs tried are ineffective for her

Treatment plan

- Ensure that she is on an adequate 'beta-blocking' dose of propranolol.
- Substitute a loop diuretic (frusemide, bumetanide) for the bendrofluazide in combination with propranolol and nifedipine.
- Try methyl dopa 250 mg tds up to 500 mg qds.
- Introduce an ACE inhibitor (capropril, enalapril) beginning with a small dose and increase as necessary – check *standing* blood pressure.

I do not think minoxidil is justified in Mrs E because of the hirsutes which may ensue.

RESISTANT HIGH BLOOD PRESSURE

> • Do you agree with this treatment plan or do you think alternative drugs should be considered?

LETTER FROM CONSULTANT TO GP

Dear John,

Thank you for your very helpful letter about this obese, asymptomatic, middle-aged hypertensive lady with a good family history who has failed to respond satisfactorily to treatment with bendrofluazide 5 mg, propranolol 240 mg and nifedipine 60 mg daily.

I have gone over her history with her and confirm that she has no symptoms; in particular there were no symptoms on direct enquiry to suggest that she may have underlying renal disease or an endocrine disturbance. I examined her carefully and like you, have found no evidence of cardiac or peripheral vascular involvement; nor does she have a renal artery murmur to suggest renal artery stenosis, or abnormality of the femoral pulse to suggest coarction. Her resting pulse rate of 60 indicates that you have given her an adequate beta-blocking dose of propranolol.

The only additional investigations I would suggest are a blood cholesterol level and an IVP (to exclude chronic asymptomatic renal disease).

The lack of satisfactory blood pressure response is likely to be due at least in part to her obesity which she has difficulty in reducing, and obviously you will have made very effort to encourage her – perhaps regular attendance at a weight-reducing club, such as 'Weight Watchers' will give her the necessary psychological motivation.

It is likely also that she will need a change to more effective drugs. In the first instance I would suggest a more potent diuretic, perhaps frusemide instead of bendrofluazide, to see if this improves blood pressure control by counteracting any fluid retention produced by the nifedipine. If this is unsuccessful a complete change of treatment would be worth considering. You could try a good old-fashioned drug like methyl-dopa, though drowsiness and fatigue might be a problem. Perhaps the best alternative drug to use would be an ACE inhibitor such as enalapril starting with a small dose, 5 mg, to exclude hypersensitivity and then progressively increasing if necessary up to 40 mg daily. Side-effects with this drug are rare but it is worth checking her standing blood pressure for postural hypertension.

Overall, I would think that the prognosis in this lady is likely to be good even if 'ideal' blood pressure control is not achieved and I have explained this to her and reassured her that I can find no complications of her hypertension. However, I have also indicated to her the desirability of trying to get better blood pressure control if we can since this will improve the future outlook even more.

Yours,

Gerald

- Do you think that the consultant's letter has adequately answered all the points raised in Dr Fry's referral letter?
- Do you think the recommended course of action is the best one for this particular patient?

OUTCOME

Mrs E was seen after consultation with GS. She was happy that nothing abnormal, apart from her high blood pressure, had been found and she accepts that further efforts should be made to control her blood pressure.

She was prescribed enalapril starting with 5 mg/day. She required two further increases to 10 mg and 15 mg/day and on the 15 mg dose her blood pressure fell to 180/100–170/90 which can be regarded as satisfactory though not 'ideal' (a blood pressure of 160/90 or below).

RESISTANT HIGH BLOOD PRESSURE

> - What complications would you be looking for in Mrs E over the course of the next 5 years?
> - What do you think will be her ultimate prognosis, say in 10–15 years?

Lessons learnt

- High blood pressure is a condition of uncertain cause and individual characteristics.
- Although there are recognized extra risks to hypertensives in general, of premature death and strokes, there are some individuals who live normally with their high blood pressures. The outlook is particularly good for overweight females.
- Since precise causes of blood pressure are unknown, treatment is pragmatic and non-response is not unusual.
- Before accepting 'resistance' check on compliance, dosage and interactions with other drugs and diet.
- Beware of causing problems for the hypertensive with side-effects from drugs used – the patient may prefer to take the risks with non-treatment.

PRACTICAL ISSUES

High blood pressure (hypertension)

- The nature and causes of the common type of hypertension are unclear and therefore management has to be pragmatic and tailored for the individual patient.
- Special attention must be paid to risky life-styles and corrective health measures should be promoted even before any medication is prescribed – for example non-smoking, weight control, regular exercise, relaxation and attention to diet.
- There are risks to life and health with continuing raised blood pressure but these are difficult to relate to the individual patient.

- Treatment is pragmatic and aims to lower the raised blood pressure with step-by-step introduction of drugs (the choices are for the physician).
- Good management demands long-term individual and personal planned care by the practice team.
- 'Resistant' high blood pressure requires an analytical approach to discover the reasons and then increase therapy with care and close observation.
- Care must always be taken to avoid making treatment worse than the disease.

Weight (obesity)

- The long-term success rates of slimming efforts are low.
- Major changes in eating habits and regular exercise are essential for success.
- Always ask how large parents and other members of the family are.

Opportunistic health promotion

- Each consultation should include discussion on health maintenance and disease prevention.
- Since specific primary prevention of hypertension is not possible, the aims have to be to diagnose it early.
- Every adult's (40 and over) blood pressure should be taken at least every 5 years and recorded.
- The case for wholesale community screening clinics and check-ups is unproven.

Communications between specialists and family doctors

- An essential part of good general practice is development of close professional relations between the family doctor and local specialists.
- Ideally the relations should develop personally as well as professionally on first name terms. Each should come to know each other's abilities and roles.
- Inevitably regular communications will have to be developed. These may be through face-to-face consultations, telephone or by letter.

SUBJECTS FOR GROUP DISCUSSION

- How to set up a long-term care programme for diagnosis and management of hypertension.
- How should the benefits of the programme be evaluated?
- Weight control – are clinics worth the effort? What evidence for success?
- What guidelines for developing understanding and relations with local specialists? What is a 'good specialist'?
- When and why should a hypertensive be referred to a specialist?

3 Breathlessness

MICHAEL G (AGED 46) – A BRICKLAYER

He has had a cough for 2 months. It is worse in the morning and he has difficulty in bringing up some sticky white sputum.
He has become breathless on effort but is able to carry out his quite heavy work.

Past history

He has consulted for winter coughs and bouts of chest wheezing for some years.

Personal history

He was born in Northern Ireland. He comes from a large family (his father was 'chesty'). He smokes about 4 ounces of rolled tobacco a week and drinks about 2–3 pints (4–6 units) of beer daily and more at weekends. His first marriage has broken up and he is living with a common-law wife (who is very caring and concerned).

Examination

A large man 6 foot and 16 stone (224 lbs), chest expansion is 2 inches. Basal wheezes on both sides.

Peak flow rate is 450 l/min

Chest X-ray is reported to be 'within normal limits'.

- What is your assessment of the case so far?
- What is normal peak flow rate for a man of his age and size?

THE GP's ASSESSMENT

A case of 'late onset asthma' or 'chronic bronchitis' or 'COAD' (chronic obstructive airways disease).

In a man of social class 3-4 who is a heavy smoker and drinker and has an unstable family background.

- What is the significance of the personal and social history in the development and progression of the condition?

MANAGEMENT BY GP

Some time has been spent with Michael G and his partner explaining the nature of his condition and likely outcome.

He has been advised to *stop* smoking, reduce his weight and cut down his drinking.

A salbutamol inhaler was prescribed and a small peak-flow meter supplied.

BREATHLESSNESS

- How can he be helped to stop smoking, reduce weight and cut down on drinking
- What is the rationale of salbutamol inhalation? What else can be tried
- What information will peak flow rates provide and how reliable are they?

Over the next two months Michael G is seen every 2 weeks:

- his cough persists
- he is short of breath
- he finds it difficult to use the inhaler and to record peak flow rates.

- You decide to refer Michael G to a consultant – why?

REFERRAL TO CONSULTANT

Dear Gerald,

Michael G (aged 46)

I seek your help for Michael G to prevent him becoming a respiratory invalid.

He is a heavy-smoking and heavy-drinking bricklayer with an unstable family background.

Over the years he has suffered from repeated lower respiratory infections.

For the past few months he has had a persistent cough, wheezing and breathlessness.

He has poor chest expansion (2 inches) for such a big man and his peak flow rate, surprisingly, is still up to 450 l/min. Chest X-ray is normal.

I have explained the importance of self-help in stopping smoking and reducing weight. I have not succeeded! There has been no response to inhalations of salbutamol, but he finds this difficult to use.

My main reason for referring him to you is the hope that you can reinforce my advice and perhaps see him a few times to achieve his cooperation.

Yours

John

- What are your comments on this referral letter?

CONSULTANT ASSESSMENT
Diagnosis

Dr Fry has quite rightly suggested that the three main diagnoses which need to be considered in this patient are:

- chronic bronchitis
- chronic obstructive airway disease
- late-onset asthma

Chronic bronchitis is defined as daily cough with sputum for at least 3 months in two consecutive years, and on this basis it is likely that Michael G fits this description. Wheezing is a frequent accompaniment though not strictly part of the definition. There may be no x-ray abnormality but sometimes distinctive changes occur.

Chronic obstructive airway disease is one of the major complications of chronic bronchitis and is due to the development of progressive emphysematous changes in the lungs. This leads to increasing ventilatory insufficiency which is reflected in a reduced peak flow rate (PFR) and an abnormal chest x-ray. Michael's PFR of 450 l/min is just within the normal range and indicates that he is unlikely to have chronic obstructive airway disease.

The diagnosis of *bronchial asthma* is made on the basis of variability of the degree of small airway obstruction, either spontaneously or as a result of treatment. However, the decision as to what constitutes adequate reversibility is sometimes difficult and may be reflected in the diagnosis of 'wheezy bronchitis' where reversibility is less than 25% and 'asthma' where it is more.

Bronchial asthma starts more frequently in childhood but it can occur at any age: the older the onset the less favourable the prognosis. Michael may have late-onset asthma but confirmation of this diagnosis will depend on showing over 25% reversibility in his small airway obstruction, either by repeated PFR measurements during his working day, or by using a bronchodilator such as his salbutamol inhaler.

Management of chronic bronchitis
General treatment

- The most important factor is to stop smoking.
- Avoid other adverse factors if possible:
    flu contacts
    going out in bad weather
    sedatives/hypnotics
    non-essential operations requiring a general anaesthetic
- Regular medical supervision:
    to detect early and treat exacerbations
    to detect and treat core pulmonale
    to encourage and support
- Education of patient and his family:
    nature and outlook of chronic bronchitis
    types of treatment available and what can and cannot be improved
    hazards of continuing to smoke

Specific treatment

- Treat infection – judge its presence by green/yellow sputum. Bacteriological examination of sputum is only of value in resistant infection. The patient could be supplied with a broad spectrum antibiotic and advised to start treatment on his own initiative if his sputum becomes green or yellow.
- Bronchodilators are always worth a trial as associated bronchospasm may be present.
- Cough medicines are of little benefit when assessed objectively but may be useful for their psychological benefits.
- Breathing exercises with chest tapping by instructed relatives may be of value.

Management of asthma

General treatment

- Educate patient and his relatives:
    the nature of asthma
    likely precipitating factors
    when to seek medical help
- Train patient to use an inhaler and the peak flow meter.
- Avoid allergens if identified.
- Treat respiratory infections promptly.
- Counselling for emotional/domestic problems.

Specific treatment

- *Bronchodilator aerosols*:
    beta-antagonists, e.g. salbutamol
    sympathomimetic – rarely used now because of side-effects, e.g. isoprenaline
    anticholinergic – worth trying if beta-agonists ineffective, e.g. ipratropium

BREATHLESSNESS

- *Methyl xanthines*, e.g. aminophylline, theophylline. The difference between the therapeutic level and toxic level is narrow so that the dose should be titrated carefully – measurement of blood levels is desirable if available. These drugs are particularly useful to prevent nocturnal asthma.
- *Cromoglycate*. This is useful when allergens can be identified. It is also useful in preventing exercise-induced asthma.
- *Steroids*. These are preferably used as aerosols to avoid side-effects. Possible hazards include candidiasis in the throat and dysphagia. Oral steroids should be reserved for the more severe attacks. It is important to watch out for the *signs of a severe attack*:
    can't lie down – too breathless
    using accessory muscles
    unable to talk
    pale and sweating
    persistent tachycardia
    pulsus paradoxus

The signs of *impending disaster* are:
    increasing cyanosis
    drowsiness and confusion
    'silent' chest
    progressive bradycardia

Patients with these signs should be admitted immediately to hospital as an acute life-threatening emergency.

LETTER FROM CONSULTANT TO GP

Dear John,

Thank you for referring this overweight bricklayer with breathlessness, wheezing and recurrent respiratory infection in winter. I note that he smokes heavily and drinks about 21 pints (42 units) of beer a week, and I note also your comment about his marital problems. You feel that it might help for me to see him and reinforce your own advice on his management.

Firstly, with reference to the diagnosis, I agree that he has either chronic bronchitis or late-onset asthma, or possibly both in the form of 'wheezy bronchitis': the normal PFR and chest X-ray would favour asthma. There is no evidence of emphysema.

I have tried to explain to him clearly and simply the nature of his lung problem and I have strongly emphasized the adverse effects of his smoking on the lungs, including the possibility of complete disablement by breathlessness due to lung damage if he persists in smoking. He was concerned about the possible adverse effect on his weight if he gave up smoking but I reassured him that this was of secondary importance and far out-weighed by the benefits of stopping the smoking. In this context also I reminded him of the calories contributed by his heavy intake of beer. I must admit I feel a bit guilty about taking away two of the comforts of his life – fortunately he didn't ask about sex!

With regard to more specific treatment, I note that he has had problems with using an inhaler. Do you think a spacer system, e.g. Volumatic or Nebuhaler might be of help, or alternatively a dry powder device (Rotahaler). If a bronchodilator alone is inadequate why not try him on beclomethasone, for a few weeks, and assess the response with PFR readings. I also think that it is always worth trying a course of cromoglycate, even if there are no obvious allergens, since I have sometimes found marked improvements in this type of chronic 'wheezy bronchitis'. Finally, the anticholinergic inhaler, ipratropium, might be useful if the other inhalers don't work too well. If he wheezes at night, it is worth trying an aminophylline tablet before he goes to bed.

I am glad you have given him a mini-peak flow meter. I have gone over it with him to confirm that he knows how to use it and I have repeated your own request to keep daily records especially before and after his various inhalers: this should tell us how effective the treatment is.

I have emphasized the need to watch out for green or yellow sputum indicating active infection, when he should have antibiotic treatment. Do you agree that it might be a good idea to supply him with a 5-day course of ampicillin or tetracycline to initiate himself if he starts to cough up infected sputum? I have explained that he should let you know as soon as convenient if

BREATHLESSNESS

he does this anyway, so that you could take over supervision of the treatment if you felt it desirable to do so.

Finally, I have arranged to review his progress in my medical clinic in 6 weeks, and I mentioned that I would particularly check up on his smoking and the records of his peak flow measurements.

Yours,

Gerald

- Your comments on this responding letter?

OUTCOME

- Michael cut his smoking by half to 2 oz a week but felt that he didn't want to do without cigarettes altogether. He was also reluctant to reduce his intake of beer in spite of the weight problem.
- He was quite good at using his peak flow meter and he did enjoy keeping records. He did not get any benefit from cromoglycate inhalations as judged by peak flow readings but did like the spacer for use with the salbutamol. He did not consider it necessary to use beclomethasone.
- He was given a supply of ampicillin to initiate treatment if his sputum became coloured and has used it quite successfully on one occasion.
- Although he was given an appointment to see the specialist again, he decided he would rather continue with his own doctor and not go to the hospital for review.

PRACTICAL ISSUES

- Chronic bronchitis is a very common condition in the UK with appreciable disability and mortality.
- The most important contributory factor is smoking and the most important treatment is to stop smoking.
- Chronic bronchitis cannot be reversed once it has become established but there is much the doctor can do to improve breathlessness, control wheezing and prevent acute exacerbations by infection.
- The doctor's constant support and encouragement in this chronic, depressing, disabling condition, and his ready availability at times of crisis, is of great psychological benefit to the patient and his family.

SUBJECTS FOR GROUP DISCUSSION

- How to instruct patient in self-use of peak flow meter?
- What is the clinical significance of differentiating between chronic bronchitis, asthma and COAD?
- How to manage the non-compliant patient?
- How can social and family circumstances affect the condition and its management?

4 Persistent dyspepsia

RICHARD S-L (AGED 40) A RESTAURATEUR

A patient with his wife and two children for 15 years. A frequent attender with bouts of 'indigestion'. The 'indigestion' has included:
bouts of nausea and abdominal distension
persistent flatulence and heartburn.

Personal history

This is his second marriage and it appears stable. His wife is supportive.

He has noted failure of erection over the past 2 months.

His early life was unhappy because his parents separated and his father drank a lot.

He smokes about 15–20 cigarettes per day. He drinks about 5 pints (10 units) of beer and 3–4 brandies daily.

Examination

Plethoric with suggestion of jaundice in conjunctivae.
Height 5 foot 9 inches
Weight 14 stone (196 lbs)

Because of obesity it is difficult to decide whether there is any enlargement of liver or spleen.

- How do you grade extent of alcohol consumption by a patient?
- What is the likely cause of his symptoms?

MANAGEMENT SO FAR

Mr S-L has been a frequent attender over the years and his symptoms have been investigated.

Blood tests have not been abnormal, including liver function tests, until now (see below).

Barium meal was reported as showing a small sliding hiatus hernia with reflux.

He has been referred to psychiatrists (two) and a gastroenterologist without much help for him.

Attempts have been made by all concerned to get him to stop drinking and smoking, without success. The most recent blood test was reported as:

		Normal range
Hb	16.1 g/dl	13–18 g/dl
MCV	103	78–98 μ^3
gamma-GT	832	10–55 u/l
AST	58	10–35 u/l
bilirubin	31	2–17 μmol/l

- What is the significance of the finding of a hiatus hernia?
- How successful is management of alcoholism?

THE GP's ASSESSMENT

Mr S-L is an alcoholic with evidence of some liver damage.

PERSISTENT DYSPEPSIA

The situation is a long-standing one and he has not been able to give up his excessive consumption of alcohol.

Now that he has become jaundiced and there is evidence of liver damage on the blood tests, he is scared and anxious to do something about it.

- What do you say to Mr and Mrs S-L?
- Why would you seek yet another specialists opinion?

REFERRAL TO CONSULTANT

Dear Gerald,

Richard S-L (Age 40)

Mr S-L has been one of my great problems over the past 15 years.

Briefly, he is suffering from effects of alcohol excess and is now at last prepared 'to do something about it!' because he has become jaundiced and I have been able to convince him that recent blood tests show liver damage. (Copies of reports are enclosed.)

I have stressed the very serious and bad prognosis if he carries on with his present level of drinking.

You are not the first consultant he has seen! He has been seen by two psychiatrists (Drs A and B) and Dr C, the gastroenterologist – you know them all. They have done their best to help him without success.

My reasons for referring him to you now are, if you agree:
- *for you to admit him to hospital, for further assessment, i.e. liver biopsy;*
- *at the same time to begin the process of detoxification and support during his withdrawal from alcohol;*
- *to arrange joint care between us to ensure long-term success.*

His wife Linda, who will attend with him, is a fine person who understands his problems and is prepared to help him as much as she can.

I believe this is a crucial time to try to prevent serious complications whilst he is in this frightened and receptive state.

Yours,

John

• What do you think of this referral letter?

CONSULTANT'S ASSESSMENT

The clinical problem is how to manage an overweight, middle-aged, hard-drinking, hard-smoking restaurateur, who has seen several specialists in the past without any benefit and who is only now apparently motivated to make some effort to help himself because of liver damage.

Diagnosis of alcoholism

The clues which may be of help in deciding when a patient can be labelled as an alcoholic are:
- family history of alcoholism (Mr S-L's father was an alcoholic);
- occupational hazards:
  - catering/drink trades (Mr S-L is a restaurateur)
  - business executives
  - commercial travellers
  - seamen
  - actors/entertainers
  - doctors!!
- history of accidents.
- work problems:
  - declining efficiency
  - unpunctuality
  - extended meal breaks
- marital problems (Mr S-L has had one divorce).

- recurrent depression.
- attempted suicide.

Clinical manifestations of alcoholism
Neuropsychiatric

- Korsakow's psychosis
- Wernicke's encephalopathy
- delirium tremens

General medical

- Cirrhosis, which may lead to:
    anorexia, flatulence, nausea, vomiting (Mr S-L has symptoms of this kind: irritable bowel syndrome is also common in alcoholics);
    bleeding tendency – spontaneous bruising
    gastrointestinal bleeding from varices/gastritis
    hepatic encephalopathy
- Anaemia:
    iron deficiency from gastrointestinal blood loss
    macrocytic from folate deficiency (Mr S-L has macrocytosis in his blood film)
- Vitamin deficiency – especially B1 and B6.
- Pancreatitis – acute and chronic.
- Cardiomyopathy.
- Peripheral neuropathy.
- Impotence (Mr S-L has this).
- Hypertension.
- Cerebellar degeneration.
- Cancer of oesophagus.

Management of alcoholism

There are two main lines of treatment:

- psychological
- treatment of physical problems

Psychological treatment

This basically involves motivation of the patient into accepting that he is an alcoholic and actively wanting to be cured. The measures which may be of help include:

- acceptance of the alcoholism:
    empathy – non-judgemental
    confrontation techniques
    optimism for future recovery
- set short-term goals – 'one day at a time'
- always involve spouse, other family members and other concerned individuals
- liaison with employer
- identify 'trigger' situations if possible – emotional or social
- Alcoholics Anonymous or other similar organizations for group therapy
- deterrent drugs:
    disulfiram
    calcium carbimide

Physical treatment
Cirrhosis

- correct nutritional deficiencies – high calorie, high protein diet with vitamin supplements, especially B1 and B6.
- vitamin K if prothrombin concentration low.

- ascites:
    reduce salt intake in food and salt-retaining drugs, e.g. NSAIDs, steroids, carbenoxolone
    diuretics
    intravenous albumen may be of temporary benefit (paracentesis should be avoided).

Pancreatitis

- pain relief.
- malabsorption managed by low-fat diet supplemented by medium-chain triglycerides.
- pancreatic extracts.

Anaemia

Treat with iron, folic acid.

Peripheral neuropathy

Treat with vitamin B1.

Wernicke's encephalopathy

May be related to B1 deficiency so treat with vitamin B1.

Korsakow's psychosis

No effective treatment available.

Cerebellar degeneration

May also be related, at least in part, to B1 deficiency so try vitamin B1.

Cardiomyopathy

No treatment required unless heart failure occurs.

LETTER FROM CONSULTANT TO GP

Dear John,

Thank you for referring Mr S-L who is a long-standing alcoholic and whom you feel may now be motivated into giving up drinking because his liver is showing signs of damage.

In the first instance, I have examined him carefully and find that, as you say, he is jaundiced, and I think he also has some other clinical manifestations of cirrhosis – his fingers are clubbed, he has a hypothenar flush and a few spider naevi on his chest and I think he has early gynaecomastia. I agree abdominal examination is difficult because of obesity but I found no convincing evidence of ascites; nor did I think his liver or spleen was enlarged. There was no evidence of liver failure – in particular no flapping tremor. The only other finding of note is evidence of chronic bronchitis attributable to his smoking. There was no evidence of cardiomyopathy or neuropathy and no memory impairment or focal cranial neurological signs to suggest either a Korsakow's psychosis or Wernicke's encephalopathy.

I have discussed the alcoholism with him in some detail and emphasized that there is no doubt about his liver damage which will get worse if he goes on drinking. As you noted, he does seem anxious and willing to have some treatment now.

I agree that it would be a good idea to admit him for a liver biopsy to assess the extent of the damage which will be of prognostic value. The other important test is a barium meal and/or gastroscopy for varices. Other tests which will be worth doing include serum amylase for pancreatitis, prothrombin concentration for potential bleeding, and faecal occult blood for actual bleeding in the GI tract. I shall also arrange for our dietician to make a thorough dietary assessment and recommend an appropriate diet with necessary supplements.

With reference to psychiatric treatment, I think there is no alternative but to seek further help. I note that this has been unsuccessful on two previous occasions but I think the outlook more hopeful now because of his motivation. His stable, loving relationship with Linda will also be of considerable help.

I agree that he will require a lot of follow-up support from you, me and the psychiatrists. I shall certainly monitor his physical progress regularly in my outpatient clinic, and I hope that my psychiatric colleagues will do the same in their clinic.

One final point – his smoking. I hope you agree that it might be better not to focus on this at present as it will take all his time and effort to stop the drinking: if this is successful we can get on to him about the smoking later.

Yours,

Gerald

OUTCOME

Mr and Mrs S-L came for a lengthy consultation with the GP.

They felt that although GS had been pleasant they were still at a loss as to what to do next.

They have heard of an eminent liver specialist in London, Dr WR and they requested yet another referral.

This was arranged (with some reluctance on the part of JF).

Dr WR, a very forthright personality, admitted Mr S-L, carried out a liver biopsy which showed evidence of early cirrhosis.

Bluntly he told S-L that his life was in his own hands. If he continued to drink 'he would be dead in 5–10 years'.

Amazingly S-L was so shaken by the eminent Dr WR that he has not drunk any alcohol since (it is now two years). He has lost weight, he has taken up regular exercise and his sexual activity is normal. Mrs S-L is very grateful.

- How usual is such an outcome?
- What is the likely prognosis over the next 5–10 years?

PRACTICAL ISSUES
What is alcoholism?

- Alcoholism is a mixture of problems and difficulties.
- The alcoholic is a vulnerable person often with many difficulties and bad past experiences.
- Alcoholism is an addiction with all the difficulties in trying to help the affected individual.
- Long-term heavy consumption of alcohol will cause serious life-threatening disorders.

Management difficulties

- The case of Mr S-L illustrates the rather untidy and unsatisfactory management by JF with difficulties in early diagnosis; difficulties in establishing good doctor–patient relations; multiple referrals to numerous specialists with none getting to grips with the problem.
- There was no evidence in this case of using non-medical community resources to help the S-L family.
- To be honest most GPs and specialists do not like having to manage alcoholics.

SUBJECTS FOR GROUP DISCUSSION

- What is the extent of the problem of alcoholism?
- How can we recognize its early features?
- How should we confront the alcoholic with his/her problems?
- What are the guidelines for care?
- Who should be involved in the management and how?
- What is the outlook for the alcoholic patient?
- What factors relate to a good or a bad prognosis?

5 Mrs 'Never Well'

MRS HILDA X (AGED 49)

Married to a bank official with one son aged 20.

Mrs X has the bulkiest (fattest) collection of records in the practice. She was allocated into the practice two years ago because her previous general practitioner had felt that 'she could do no more for her!'.

Past history

The story goes back 20 years. Soon after the birth of her son – a difficult pregnancy and a stormy labour with forceps extraction after 16 hours – Mrs X had begun to experience lower abdominal pains. These went on and on and involved repeated investigations and repeated referrals to many specialists. A normal appendix was removed 15 years ago and other organs were reported as normal.

She has had barium meals, barium enemas, cholecystograms, endoscopies at both ends of her gastrointestinal tract, and intravenous urograms.

She has seen gynaecologists and had two laparoscopies and many, many urine and blood tests. No organic disorders have been detected. She has been seen by psychiatrists and psychotherapists.

Present problems

Mrs X continues to attend frequently and she continues to complain bitterly of constant burning in her lower abdomen.

She and her husband are sure there must be something wrong somewhere and are blaming the medical profession for being unable to diagnose and cure her.

Bowels and micturition are normal.

She still menstruates regularly and complains of premenstrual tension.

Examination

Was remarkably unremarkable.
There is an appendicectomy scar.
She is overweight but nothing abnormal to feel.

- What do you make of this story?
- Why has she had so many investigations and referrals?
- How would *you* have managed her?

MANAGEMENT

Mr X was seen alone and an attempt was made to put a psychopathological explanation to him. He did not accept this.

He asks for one more independent opinion. Weakening, it is agreed that this should be the last one!

- What else might you do?

Personal and family history

Mrs X has always been 'nervy' as was her mother, but has been worse since her one and only pregnancy. She has had bouts of depression and, from her notes, it seems that she has been prescribed most of the known antidepressants and tranquillizers over the past 20 years – none has helped her for any time, nor did the consultations with psychiatrists and psychotherapists.

The marital situation is fragile. Mrs X has been uninterested in sex since her pregnancy and this has made her husband fed up and devoting his spare time interests elsewhere.

Mrs X would like to work part time but she spends a day or two each week in bed because of her symptoms.

Their son, now 20, has been a worry to them for the past 5 years. He left school unprepared for his future, has not held a job down for more than a few months at a time, has been drinking excessively and experimenting with drugs.

THE GPs ASSESSMENT

Mrs X has a 'fat-folder syndrome', it has been labelled otherwise over the years as 'hysteria', 'somatization syndrome', 'nervous bowel', 'irritable bowel syndrome', 'spastic colon' and probably many others.

She has used up much doctor time and cost the health service a lot.

No one in the past seems to have been able to help her and there is no reason why you or anyone else will succeed in the future.

Faced with unpleasantness if you refuse, a further referral is agreed.

- What do you say to Mr *and* Mrs X?
- What do you plan to do after she has been seen by the specialist?

SECOND OPINIONS IN INTERNAL MEDICINE

REFERRAL TO CONSULTANT

Dear Gerald,

Mrs Hilda X (Aged 49)

I am sorry to burden you with Mrs X but I seek your help and cooperation.

She has a 20 year + history of chronic abdominal pains. She must have seen upwards of 40 doctors over this time and had hundreds of investigations. I will not list them all (but will send you the reports if you wish). Needless to say no abnormalities have been detected.

I have only known the family for the past two years and have resisted referring her for any investigations or opinion.

I am faced with a near crisis situation. Both Mr and Mrs X are sure that there is something wrong somewhere and have become very anti-doctor and I imagine would be only too pleased to sue or complain given a cause or reason.

So I have weakened to arrange a consultation with you. If you agree, I ask you to reinforce my policies:
- *to confirm that you cannot find any organic cause for her symptoms*
- *to agree that further investigations are not necessary*
- *to provide them with some feasible explanation and suggest that she will have to live with her symptoms which hopefully will improve in time*

Yours apologetically,

John

- What is your opinion of this referral letter?

CONSULTANT ASSESSMENT

The clinical problem is a 49-year-old lady with a 20-year history of apparently intractable burning lower abdominal pain which has persisted in spite of seeing many specialists and having a large number of investigations, including two laparoscopies.

There are many causes of chronic abdominal pain and diagnosis may be very difficult in spite of the expertise of GPs, physicians, surgeons, gynaecologists and psychiatrists. The first step in diagnosis is to consider the possible causes:

Abdominal	• peptic ulcer diseases
	    oesophagitis
	    gastric ulcer
	    duodenal ulcer
	• chronic cholecystitis
	• chronic pancreatitis
	• chronic liver congestion (heart failure)
	• inflammatory bowel disease
	    ulcerative colitis
	    Crohn's disease
	• mesenteric ischaemia
	• irritable bowel syndrome

Gynaecological	• pelvic inflammatory disease • uterine and ovarian tumours

Extra-abdominal	• metabolic
	    uraemia
	    porphyria
	    Addison's disease
	    lead poisoning

Neurogenic	• degenerative arthritis spine • peripheral neuritis • tabes dorsalis
Psychogenic	• anxiety • depression

In the great majority of cases the diagnosis is made on the basis of a detailed and careful history, bearing in mind the five important features in dealing with abdominal pain:

- site of the pain
- character of the pain
- aggravating factors
- relieving factors
- associated features

Although Mrs X has been assessed many times, and her 'Fat Folder Syndrome' can be intimidating, I think it important to explore the history carefully with her once again and also carry out a thorough clinical examination. Although it is very unlikely to lead to any new revelations which may have been missed by other specialists, at the very least it will show Mrs X that she has been taken seriously, and, hopefully, may provide the further reassurance that such patients are so often desperately seeking.

Analysis of the GP's findings
Gynaecological history

She had a difficult pregnancy and a 'stormy labour'. This would suggest the possibility of underlying chronic pelvic disease: I'm sure, however, that this will have been satisfactorily excluded by the gynaecologists she has seen previously. Additionally, the normal periods would exclude any serious gynaecological disease.

Site of the pain

The pain is lower abdominal, which suggests that the origin may be in the colon, in the bladder or in the pelvis. One other possibility which should always be kept in mind is referred pain from the thoraco-lumbar spine.

Character of the pain

The pain is described as 'burning': this raises the possibility of a causalgia-type pain due to nerve root irritation. The duration of the pain would obviously exclude an acute cause such as herpes zoster but chronic conditions which may cause long-standing causalgia include nerve injury from wounds/incisions and nerve root irritation from degenerative changes in the spine. If Mrs X has not seen an orthopaedic specialist before then this is something that might be worth considering also.

However, psychogenic pain can take many different forms and 'burning' pain may well be one of them.

Normal investigations

The normal barium meal, barium enema, cholecystogram, urogram and endoscopies will have satisfactorily excluded organic disease of the gastrointestinal tract, gall-bladder and kidneys.

Psychological factors

There is no doubt from Dr Fry's letter that Mrs X (as well as Mr X) are under considerable stress and anxiety, but whether this is a causal factor or a result of the chronic pain may be difficult to decide – it may of course be both!

CONSULTANT'S LETTER TO THE GP

Dear John,

Thank you for referring this unfortunate 49-year-old lady with apparently intractable abdominal pain for the last 20 years. I note how thoroughly she has been investigated but all to no avail, and I can appreciate your problem in managing her. I can think of two other ladies attending my clinic at present with identical symptoms, not to mention a large number in the past who will no doubt have moved on to other specialist colleagues in their search for the answer to their problems.

The first thing which I have done, which I consider essential in this type of problem, is to take a detailed and unhurried history of her abdominal and other symptoms, which I'm sure she appreciated (though I wouldn't dare to say the same appreciation was felt by the other patients who were waiting to see me in the clinic!). As I have indicated, she complains of constant burning pain in the lower abdomen which she maintains lasts all day and occurs every day. There are no obvious aggravating or relieving factors apart from a rather grudging admission that the pain tends to be a bit worse when she is under stress. There is no associated diarrhoea which is against any inflammatory bowel disease: the absence of postprandial diarrhoea would also make chronic mesenteric ischaemia unlikely. There is no obvious abnormality of her stools: they are not bulky or offensive as in chronic pancreatitis, no blood or pus as in inflammatory disease due to diverticulitis and no pellet or ribbon appearance as in irritable bowel syndrome. There were no associated urinary symptoms and no relationship between the pain and her periods to suggest a gynaecological cause. She does, however, admit that she gets a lot of wind and abdominal distension, though not particularly related to the pain which is there most of the time.

I examined her carefully. I agree that she has no abnormal masses or palpable viscera but she was slightly tender over the lower abdomen, more so in the iliac fossae than in the suprapubic region. One other interesting finding, which may or may not be relevant, is that she does have evidence of lumbar osteoarthritis with limited forward flexion and lateral flexion, of her spine, especially to the right. Additionally, she thought that the lower abdominal pain might have been a bit worse during the lateral flexion of the spine. I could not find any neurological abnormality, especially no sensory changes in the abdominal wall or evidence of peripheral neuropathy. The cardiovascular and respiratory systems were also normal.

In conclusion, like many of the other specialists who have seen Mrs X, I can find no evidence of any organic intra-abdominal disease, and I have reassured her as strongly as I can about this; in particular I have stressed that she does not have cancer. In this respect it is interesting that she did admit, as many of my similar patients have done in the past, that this is one of the conditions she dreads most, especially as her mother and one of her sisters both died of bowel cancer in their fifties. I hope that this reassurance – which I am sure will have been given to Mrs X many times before – will be of some help, at least temporarily. I think that there are undoubtedly some features of irritable bowel syndrome, and with this diagnosis in mind, I have tried to explain to her that her pain is due to muscle spasm in the bowel as a result of tension and anxiety. I further explained that tension in the mind as a result of stress can produce similar tension, or spasm, in the muscles. I don't know whether this explanation will convince Mrs X as, no doubt she has heard it many times before, but I remain hopeful. I have encouraged her to stick more rigidly to her high-fibre diet, which she admitted she had not been doing.

I do not think any further investigations would be of value – she has had too many already! Perhaps, one test we could do if it has not been done for a while is an X-ray of her spine for degenerative changes: if these are substantial how would you feel about trying her on a spinal support to see if this helps?

I have not made a further appointment to see her again, but if you feel this would be of any help to you at any time please do not hesitate to contact me again.

Yours

Gerald

OUTCOME

One year later the situation is worse:

- Mrs X still suffers from her usual symptoms.
- Mr X is threatening to leave home (he has a 'girl friend').
- Son has been in trouble with the police and is on probation on a drug charge.

PRACTICAL ISSUES

- As well as taking up much of the doctor's time these patients also use up much of the investigative resources – how to control these?
- Were all the many referrals really necessary?
- Would a different plan of management have been better and if so, what?

SUBJECTS FOR GROUP DISCUSSION

- Put together the features of this syndrome.
- What is its frequency and prognosis?
- How best to cope with these patients?
- How to achieve a common policy with specialist colleagues?

6 Headaches

JOAN E (AGED 57) UNMARRIED LEGAL SECRETARY

Recently moved into the district and consults for the first time.

Reason for consultation is a request for a prescription of ampoules of dihydroergotamine mesylate 1 mg for self-injection. Her story is that she has suffered from 'terrible' headaches for over 30 years and the injections are the only treatment that has helped her.

Past history

Headaches are described as 'severe pressure'. Sited over maxillary regions and occiput. May last for a few days and are accompanied by malaise and nausea. No history of visual disturbances or nasal or eye discharge.

Her large bundle of medical records show that she has been seen and been investigated by many specialists, including neurologists, rhinolaryngologists, general physicians and psychiatrists.

Her treatment included analgesics, antidepressants, carbamezepine and benzodiazepines. She has had her sinuses washed out and her nasal septum resected. Hypnotherapy has been tried.

The treatments appear to relieve her symptoms for a while and then recur.

Her previous doctor suggested that she try ergotamine. Tablets were not very helpful but an injection of dihydroergotamine mesylate (1 mg) was effective and continues to be. Her method is to inject herself as soon as she feels the headache coming on. She uses 3–4 ampoules a week.

Family history

An aunt suffered from migraine.

Personal history

She lived with her widowed mother until she died. She has no siblings. She is a specialized legal secretary. She has no personal or financial worries. Has never smoked and does not drink alcohol.

Examination

A pleasant and relaxed person with no obvious suggestions of any psychiatric disorders.
There are no abnormal physical signs.
BP 135/65.
Peripheral pulses all present.
Wears spectacles at work.

- What is the rationale of using ergotamine?
- What do you think of the treatment in this case?
- What is your assessment of the case so far?

MANAGEMENT

Following a lengthy discussion with Miss E on the nature of her condition and the treatment it is agreed that you contact her previous doctor (Dr M) and arrange to see her the next day.

You phone Dr M and he states that he has known Joan E for about 25 years and confirms her story. He does not believe her to be neurotic or unstable, on the contrary, she is a most reliable and steady person. He has tried to stop the ergotamine but she has resisted this.

- What else would you do?

THE GP's ASSESSMENT

Joan E's story is not typical of migraine.

Ergotamine may have serious side-effects when taken long term.

Not very happy to continue to prescribe ampoules for self-administration.

She will be unhappy if she is not given the prescription.

- What explanation do you give her?
- Why would you seek her agreement for a referral?

REFERRAL TO CONSULTANT

Dear Gerald,

Miss Joan E (57)

Miss E is a new patient who presents a tricky problem for me. She has suffered for over 30 years with troublesome headaches for which she has been seen by many consultants and had many investigations. None appears to have revealed any organic abnormalities.

A diagnosis of 'sinusitis' led to sinus washouts and SMR operations on her nasal septum.

Past medications have included analgesics, antidepressants, tranquillizers and beta-blockers.

For the past 5 years she has been injecting herself with dihydroergotamine mesylate 1 mg p.r.n. She uses 3–4 per week.

I have just met her for the first time and she wants me to give her a further prescription for the ergotamine.

My reason for referring her to you rather urgently is to get your support and approval for my continuing her medication.

She appears to be emotionally stable and not addicted to the drug.

From her history I an not convinced that she has 'migraine', even of the most atypical variety, but it does seem that the injections of dihydroergotamine are specific in their effects.

What is your advice?

Yours,

John

- What is your opinion of this referral letter?

CONSULTANT'S ASSESSMENT

The clinical problem is how to manage a much-investigated lady of 57 with a long-standing history of severe headache not typical of migraine who appears to have become dependent on ergotamine.

Causes of headache

The two most commonest causes of headache are psychogenic ('tension' headache) and migraine. Other causes include:

raised intracranial pressure
vascular disorders
- hypertension
- temporal arteritis
- subarachnoid haemorrhage

local disease
- sinusitis
- eye disease
- cervical spondylosis
- bone disease e.g. Paget's disease, myeloma

The diagnosis of a headache is based primarily on the symptoms. Clinical examination is unlikely to help if the history does not indicate the cause, and investigation is even less likely to reveal the answer in the presence of a negative history and examination. The diagnostic features of some common types of headache are shown in Table 6.1.

Treatment of migraine

The treatment of migraine is based on general measures, treatment of the acute attack and prevention of attacks.

General measures

- Patient education.
- Avoidance of trigger factors.
- Loop diuretic in premenstrual week if migraine occurs at this time.
- Discourage oestrogens for both birth control and menopausal symptoms.
- Avoid vasodilator drugs.

Treatment of an acute attack

Ergot preparations
- oral
- suppository
- aerosol
- sublingual
- injection

Combined preparations
(useful in controlling the vomiting as well as the headache)
- Migraleve
  buclizine
  paracetamol
  codeine
- Migravess
  metoclopramide
  aspirin
- Migril
  ergotamine
  cyclizine
  caffeine

N.B. Maxolon (metoclopramide) is also of value in the acute attack because it can reduce the nausea and vomiting and can also expedite absorption of any analgesic used (gastric stasis occurs in an attack of migraine and retards drug absorption).

Toxicity of ergot preparations

Although ergot toxicity is rare in the treatment of migraine it is important not to exceed the recommended doses, e.g. maximum dose of ergotamine is 6 mg in a single attack or 10 mg in one week. The side-effects are:

- nausea/vomiting
- abdominal pain
- muscle cramps
- gangrene
- mental disturbance
- withdrawal symptoms may occur

Table 6.1 Diagnostic features of common headaches

	'Tension'	Migraine	R.I.P.	Hypertension	Cervical spondylosis
Character	'pressure', 'weight' 'tight band' other bizarre descriptions	throbbing	throbbing, bursting	throbbing	aching, burning
Site	often vertex 'all over' any site	hemicranial	frontal with supratentorial tumours; occipital with posterior fossa tumours	occipital (temporal in arteritis)	occipital
Duration	hours, days, weeks	hours, occasionally a day or two	constant, worse at night or on waking, straining, coughing, bending	constant, worse at night or on waking, straining, coughing, bending	minutes or hours
Triggers	anxiety	mental stress, menstruation, alcohol, foodstuffs	constant, worse at night or on waking, straining, coughing, bending	constant, worse at night or on waking, straining, coughing, bending	
Associations	left mammary pain, palpitations, 'can't breathe deeply', tremor	visual upset (teichopsia) nausea/vomiting – relieves headache	blurred vision,- vomiting – doesn't relieve headache	vomiting when severe	dizziness related to head movement

CONSULTANT'S LETTER TO THE GP

Dear John,

Thank you for referring this lady with long-standing 'terrible headaches'. I note that she seems to have become dependent on her injections of ergot and you are naturally worried about the possibility of long-term side-effects.

In the first instance I have discussed her symptoms with her in some detail and I think that she probably gets more than one type of headache. Certainly the headache that seems to be giving her most trouble at present is the 'severe pressure' which she sites over the occipital area and sometimes, she admitted, over the vertex, and this may last for days at a time.

I have little doubt that this is 'tension headache'. Although she maintains that she does not have any worries I am sure that there is quite a lot of strain at her work and I would suspect that she does have one or two personal problems. Regrettably I did not have time to probe this further but no doubt the psychiatrist she has seen previously would have gone into this in some detail.

On direct enquiry, however, it appears that she also gets attacks of throbbing headache over the parietal area on occasions associated with nausea. She told me that this type of headache had been more frequent prior to her menopause. I understand that she was put on ergotamine originally for this headache but has been using it subsequently for her other headaches as well. I have tried to explain to her the distinction between the two types of headache and suggested that she uses the injections only for the throbbing headache because of the likelihood of serious side-effects.

I have considered two other possible contributory factors in relation to her headache – maxillary sinusitis and cervical spondylosis. She does have some tenderness over the maxillary antra and I am arranging an X-ray of her sinuses; it is a long time since she has attended the ENT department and she may have developed some pathology now. There is also some restriction of neck movements suggesting cervical spondylosis. I wonder if you think it might be worth trying her with a collar for a time.

With regard to treatment of the headache I note that psychotropic drugs and hypnotherapy have not really helped. If she can manage to separate the migrainous type of headache from the 'tension headache' then perhaps a trial of pizotifen in full dosage of 6 mg in 24 hours may help as I have found it a good prophylactic in migraine. As far as the ergotamine injections are concerned, which she is currently taking in a dose of 3–4 mg a week, I don't think that she will get into trouble as the maximum recommended dose of ergotamine in the British National Formulary is 8–10 mg/week.

One final thought; with this type of problem one is tempted to try a placebo injection of saline if she can be persuaded it is a new and effective injection for her kind of headache. It would be interesting to assess her response. What do you think?

Yours,

Gerald

OUTCOME

Five years later Joan E is now 62 and has retired from work. She says she 'does not know how she had time to go to work before!' as she is so busy with her church work and voluntary services for the elderly. She is happy and well.

Her headaches still occur two or three times a month. She is continuing to give herself injections of ergotamine. There are no apparent ill effects of its long-term use.

She consults JF three or four times a year for repeat prescriptions of ergotamine, disposable syringes and needles.

PRACTICAL ISSUES

- The difficulties in diagnosing and managing chronic headache in practice are great.
- Multiple referrals to a wide variety of specialists usually denote that none of them is any better than the GP in coping with the patient's problems.
- Starting a patient on self-medication (injection) of a potentially harmful drug (ergotamine) is fraught with difficulties and dangers.
- Accept that the natural history of many common chronic conditions is surprising and instructive to the doctor and he must be prepared to learn from each such experience and regularly analyse his records.

SUBJECTS FOR GROUP DISCUSSION

- Epidemiology of headache in the community, i.e. prevalence, nature, course and outcome.
- Early features of a serious type of headache that requires urgent specialist intervention.
- Management of conditions that do not fit text-book descriptions.
- The range of self-care and the doctor's responsibilities.
- Personal, family and social factors that may produce chronic headache.
- Dealing with a patient who insists on continuing with a potentially dangerous drug.

7 Swollen legs

CHARLOTTE F (AGED 76)

A housewife living with a retired husband and an unmarried daughter. Moved into the practice about one year ago, and her records have only recently arrived.

She complained of painful swollen legs and breathlessness.

Examination

She is grossly overweight 13 stone 2 pounds, 5 feet 2 inches. Considerable tight swelling of legs below both knees. No varicose veins seen.

Liposclerosis of lower third of legs. Both knees are arthritic. Heart size could not be assessed. Pulse rate 76 regular. BP 150/84

- What are the likely causes of her swollen legs?
- What do you do next?

Past history

You then go through her past records (of her previous GP, for 30 years).

She had a subtotal hysterectomy in 1950 and a vulvectomy in 1973 for leukoplakia. These are the BP readings from 1955 on:

In 1955 – 170/100 – treated with phenobarbitone and theobromine
1965 – 210/120 and 180/110 – no treatment
1975 – 180/90 – when she was prescribed propranolol 40 mg daily
1980 – 210/120 – still on propranolol, now 80 mg daily
1985 – 190/100 – still on propranolol

Seen by me in 1986 her BP was 150/80 and she had not bothered to take propranolol for past 3 months. On trial without any medication her BP remained at 150/80 to 170/90.

- What are your comments on the course of BP levels?
- What do you think of the past management?
- What would you do about the BP now?

RECENT MANAGEMENT

Mrs F is advised to try and lose weight by dieting. Her weight does not go down.

She is ordered elastic support stockings and prescribed diuretics (bendrofluazide 5 mg and then frusemide 40 mg daily) with no reduction of leg swelling.

She is fed up and wants to see a specialist!

THE GP's ASSESSMENT

Mrs F has severe leg swelling unresponsive to treatment.

It is most likely to be the result of old venous/lymphatic occlusion of legs, possibly following her pelvic operations.

She is unhappy.

SWOLLEN LEGS

It is unlikely that her leg swelling will be reduced without drastic measures such as weight reduction and graduated pressure stockings.

In such a situation a referral to GS might defuse the situation.

- What do you say to Mrs F?
- What expectations do you give her?

REFERRAL TO CONSULTANT

Dear Gerald,

Mrs Charlotte F (Aged 76)

Mrs F is a problem for me. She has had swollen legs for many years. She is overweight and cannot reduce it.

In the past she had raised BP but now it appears that her BP is within normal limits without treatment. I can find no evidence of cardiac failure but I have not investigated this aspect.

It is likely that she has old deep vein thrombosis (she had a hysterectomy in 1950 and vulvectomy in 1973 for leukoplakia).

I have tried support stockings and diuretics (bendrofluazide 5 mg and frusemide 40 mg daily) with no improvement.

She is unhappy that I have been unable to work a miracle!

I am referring her mainly to seek your support to inform her that there is not much more to be done, unless she loses weight, or can you suggest something more?

Yours,

John

- What critique of this letter?

CONSULTANT'S ASSESSMENT

The clinical problem is painful swollen legs, breathlessness and obesity.

The causes of bilateral swelling of the legs which need to be considered are:

- heart failure
- nephrotic syndrome
- hepatic disease
- local obstruction

If local obstruction is a possible diagnosis as seems to be the case in this patient, then the causes of such obstruction include:

Primary	• congenital
	• Milroy's disease
Secondary	• recurrent lymphangitis
	• malignancy direct invasion
	• lymph node pressure

Analysis of the GP's findings

The relevant features in Dr Fry's clinical presentation which need to be discussed are:

- the breathlessness
- the type of oedema
- the significance of the hypertension

Breathlessness

This could be a manifestation of left ventricular failure or simply due to obesity. It would be important to know whether Mrs F's breathlessness has been progressive and whether it has resulted in orthopnoea or, more seriously, paroxysmal nocturnal dyspnoea: this type of progress would undoubtedly suggest left ventricular failure. The relevance of this to the oedema is that long-standing left ventricular failure can lead to right ventricular failure and oedema. It will be necessary, therefore, to check whether Mrs F has any evidence of left ventricular failure such as a gallop rhythm and/or basal pulmonary crepitations.

Oedema

The distinction between venous oedema and lymphatic oedema is based on several criteria:

- venous oedema is pitting, lymphatic oedema is not;
- lymphatic oedema may have a sharp cut-off point midway along the dorsum of the foot;
- the skin overlying lymphatic oedema is coarsened and may resemble orange peel.

If the oedema is *lymphatic* then the lymph nodes will need to be assessed in Mrs F's groin as well as the possibility of any intra-pelvic or intra-abdominal malignancy.

If the oedema is *venous* then the distinction must be made between a generalized cause, such as right ventricular failure or nephrotic syndrome, and localized obstruction. Right ventricular failure would be indicated by cyanosis, distended neck veins, and a congested liver: nephrotic syndrome is suggested by peri-orbital oedema and ascites, and these signs should be sought when Mrs F is examined.

As far as localized oedema is concerned Dr Fry has already indicated that there are no visible varicose veins so this cause is excluded. The other major cause of oedema due to venous obstruction is venous thrombosis and Dr Fry's view is that this is likely to be the cause in Mrs F. She is complaining of painful legs, and if the pain is in the calf or along the femoral canal in the medial part of the thigh, then the likelihood of venous thrombosis is increased, though bilateral involvement is perhaps unlikely. However, the only definitive way of deciding a diagnosis of deep vein thrombosis is by phlebography.

One other important cause of leg oedema that tends to be overlooked is whether it could be drug-induced. The drugs in common use which are associated sometimes with fluid retention include:

- Vasodilators for hypertension:
    hydrallazine
    nifedipine
    minoxidil
- Non-steroidal anti-inflammatory drugs
- Steroids

Hypertension

The relevance of the hypertension is its role in causing left ventricular failure. The blood pressure recorded since 1955 has shown a consistent increase until 1985 though the last measurement, in Dr Fry's referral letter, was normal on no hypertensive treatment. Assessment of target organ damage would be an important indication of the severity and significance of the long-standing hypertension. This assessment would include:

Heart	• LV enlargement on examination
	• X-ray evidence of cardiomegaly
	• ECG evidence of LV hypertrophy
Kidney	• proteinuria
	• blood urea/serum creatinine levels
	• IVP (possibly)
Arteries	• clinical evidence of arteriosclerosis in foot pulses and fundal arterioles

SWOLLEN LEGS

CONSULTANT'S LETTER TO THE GP

Dear John,

Thank you for referring this elderly lady with apparently intractable swollen legs. I note that you think the most likely cause is old deep vein thrombosis probably following her pelvic operations in 1950 and 1973.

I have gone into her history with her in some detail and think that your suggestion of venous thrombosis is a good one, since she told me that she can remember having a painful swollen leg following the operation in 1973. She thinks that the swelling of both legs really started from about this time.

I have examined her carefully. As far as her legs are concerned I think that she has a mixture of lymphatic and venous oedema since there is some pitting of the ankles and feet although not enough to account for all the swelling. There was no tenderness over the saphenous vein in the calf or over the femoral canal so I do not think she has active thrombophlebitis. I could not feel any abnormal lymph nodes in the groins. I did not do a pelvic examination. I found no evidence of either right or left ventricular failure and there are no signs of nephrotic syndrome or hepatic disease.

I would agree with you that old deep vein thrombosis is likely to be a significant factor in causing Mrs F's swollen legs but lymphoedema is also in part to blame though I can't find a primary cause for this – in particular, there is no evidence of any malignancy.

I do not really think that any special investigations are going to help in the management. Phlebography might confirm venous thrombosis but it will not influence Mrs F's treatment. Even if she developed an acute thrombosis I would be reluctant to give her anticoagulant therapy because of the considerable risk of bleeding at her age.

With regard to treatment of her legs I have very little to add to what you are doing already – elastic supports, which I think are the most important part of the treatment, and diuretics to control what fluid there is in the legs. I have also encouraged her to keep her legs up on a stool whenever she is sitting down. If you feel it would be of any help at any time I would be quite happy to take her into hospital for a few days to try some more intensive diuretic therapy under close supervision which would certainly get rid of any excess fluid retention. At the same time we could try using our special intermittent pressure 'boot' which we use in resistant oedema: it is often quite effective in providing temporary relief of the swelling.

One final point about her obesity. I know it would be good for her to lose some weight, but as she has so far failed to do so in spite of constant pleading, I really feel that any further advice is unlikely to be heeded and I have not therefore given her any – I think her food is one of her last remaining pleasures in life anyway.

In conclusion, I have reassured Mrs F that your management of her condition is exactly what I would do myself and that all the necessary treatment is being given. I am sure that she felt a lot happier after the consultation with me.

Yours sincerely,

Gerald

OUTCOME

Three years later Mrs F continues to live with her daughter. Unfortunately Mr F died a year ago from carcinoma of the prostate.

She is much less mobile. Her legs are still swollen and the left is ulcerated and is being managed by the district nurse.

She found the support stockings very uncomfortable and has not worn them. Diuretics had no effect on the swelling. Her weight has gone up. BP remains 150/80.

Mrs F accepts her condition and does not complain.

PRACTICAL ISSUES

- There are many 'non-curable' situations in medicine such as the case of Mrs F.
- An important lesson is that sometimes one should not try too hard with uncomfortable (support stockings) and potentially risky (long-term diuretics) measures.
- Another important lesson is to note the return of pressure to normal readings 20 years after it had been noted to be high. This is by no means unusual in elderly persons and it is reasonable to withdraw antihypertensive therapy sometimes to see whether the BP remains low.

SUBJECTS FOR GROUP DISCUSSION

- Epidemiology of swollen legs – how frequent in the community and cause?
- What is the course and outcome of cases such as Mrs F and what risks and complications?
- How can function and independence be maintained and promoted in old fat ladies with swollen legs?
- Are there any preventive measures that may be used now?

8 Multiple Joint Pains

LESLIE H (AGED 69) RETIRED GREENGROCER

A long history of occupational dermatitis of hands which eventually became widespread.

'Acute R. frozen shoulder' in January which did not respond to injection of local steroids.

Two weeks later presented with 'R. tennis elbow' but in a few days it became obvious this was a wrong diagnosis as he had an acute arthritis of the elbow.

Over the next month he developed painful swellings of wrists, knees and L. temporo-mandibular joint.

He was very unwell and went to bed. The blood test results were as follows:

Hb	14.6 g/dl (normal 13–18 g/dl)
ESR	9 mm/hour (normal 5-15 mm/h)
Rheumatoid factor	positive

MANAGEMENT

Treated with aspirin and other NSAIDs and finally a short course of oral steroids was given.

Improvements minimal – he was able to walk and go out but 3 months from onset he had generalized painful joints.

> - What are the possible diagnoses?
> - Comment on the management so far.

THE GP's ASSESSMENT

A well-known patient who does not complain readily but who is suddenly disabled with an acute polyarthritis.
Although the ESR is low the rheumatoid factor is positive.
He has not responded to salicylates and NSAIDs and even to a short course of steroids.
You decide to seek specialist advice.

> - What is unusual in this clinical presentation?
> - What do you say to Mr and Mrs H?

REFERRAL TO CONSULTANT

Dear Gerald,

Leslie H (aged 69)
Mr H is a retired self-employed greengrocer who has always been very active physically. Over the past 3 months he has become severely disabled with an acute polyarthritis. He has a long history of dermatitis which I thought was occupational, this has improved since he retired. I have treated him with:

- *a period of bed rest*
- *aspirin up to 2.4 g daily*
- *indomethacin up to 100 mg daily*
- *a 10 day course of prednisolone 20 mg daily*

He has not improved very much, but is now able to walk with discomfort.
   Surprisingly his ESR is only 9 mm/hour but his rheumatoid factor is reported as positive.

MULTIPLE JOINT PAINS

I am uncertain of the exact diagnosis and even less certain about what to do next. May we have your help.

Yours,

John

- What else would you put into this letter?
- How would you arrange a consultation and where?
- What are your expectations from the consultation?

CONSULTANT'S ASSESSMENT
Diagnosis

The causes of recurrent polyarthritis over a period of 3 months which need to be considered in the patient include:

- rheumatoid arthritis
- psoriatic arthropathy
- gout
- collagen disease
- Reiter's syndrome
- systemic disease:
    ulcerative colitis/Crohn's disease
    malignancy
    amyloidosis
    sarcoidosis

Significance of positive rheumatoid factor

Rheumatoid factor is usually present in:
- rheumatoid arthritis (80%)
- polyarthritis nodosa
- sarcoidosis

Rheumatoid factor is usually absent in:
- SLE
- psoriasis
- inflammatory bowel disease
- rheumatoid arthritis (20%)

Other investigations to help diagnosis
X-ray

X-ray of the joints is the simplest test

rheumatoid	• juxta-articular osteoporosis
	• narrow joint spaces
	• marginal and cystic erosions
	• dislocations/joint deformity
psoriasis	• affects terminal phalanges fingers/toes
	• metacarpal/metatarsal heads may disappear
	• spine/sacro-iliac joints may be affected
gout	• first metatarso-phalangeal joint usually affected
	• subarticular cysts
	• 'punched-out' marginal erosions
Reiter's	• local periostitis
	• sacro-iliitis
Ulcerative colitis/	• sacro-iliitis
Crohn's	• ankylosing spondylitis
	• (changes in bowel on barium enema)

Blood tests

Gout:	• increased uric acid
Sarcoidosis:	• serum calcium
	• serum globulin

MULTIPLE JOINT PAINS

Collagen screen:	• SLE – antinuclear antibodies invariable • DNA-binding invariable
HLA-typing:	• rheumatoid – DR4 DW4 • psoriasis – B27 BW38 • Reiter's – B27

(The ESR is too non-specific to be of any diagnostic help.)

MANAGEMENT OF RHEUMATOID ARTHRITIS
Acute phase

General	• bed rest • immobilization of painful joints • heat/wax baths to relieve pain and stiffness • exercises after subsidence of acute pain
Drugs	• aspirin • NSAIDs, e.g. indomethacin, naprosyn, ibuprofen

Long-term treatment
General

- Education of patient and family: nature of condition, prognosis, what treatment can and cannot do.
- Iron if anaemic (GI blood loss from treatment).
- Treatment of depression – drugs only if severe.
- Constant support/encouragement from GP.

Physiotherapy

- Exercises to maintain joint/muscle function.
- Advice on correct use of joint to avoid strain.
- Hydrotherapy to encourage movement.
- Heat to relieve pain and spasm.

Occupational Therapy

- Splinting to preserve function.
- Assessment of activity and best way to accomplish tasks.
- Appliances/gadgets for household tasks.
- Special fixtures/fittings in kitchen and bathroom.

Social services

Home nurses

- Help with working/bathing.
- Check and advise on drug treatment.
- Assess and arrange for aids.
- Encourage and support.

Social worker

- Advice on finance.
- Advice on welfare rights: attendance allowance, mobility allowance, heating allowance.
- Arrange home helps.
- Arrange meals-on-wheels.
- Organize attendance at day centre.
- Organize 'night-sitters' if required.
- Assess housing requirements

Drug treatments

- Aspirin – 4 to 6 g/day
- NSAIDs
- Gold indications:
    active progressive disease in spite of other treatment
    nodules and high titres of rheumatoid factor
    extra-articular disease: episcleritis, pleurisy/pericarditis, vasculitis, pulmonary involvement, polyneuritis, myositis

Administration

Gold is given by i.m. injections, 50 mg weekly for 2 to 3 months, then as required (always use a test dose first).

Side-effects:
- Rashes
- Mouth ulcers
- Nephrotic syndrome
- Pancytopenia
- Enterocolitis

Penicillamine

Indications – as for gold.
Administration – 125–250 mg orally daily increasing up to 1 g/day.
Side effects – as for gold but also loss of taste.

Steroids

Indications:
- severe exacerbations unresponsive to rest and NSAIDs
- persistent disabling disease in a young mother or breadwinner unresponsive to other treatment
- severe extra-articular disease

Dosage:
- start with 20–30 mg prednisolone a day but reduce this to a minimum, preferably not more than 7.5 mg/day, as soon as possible to avoid side-effects

Side-effects:
- fluid retention 7 oedema
- hypertension
- diabetes
- peptic ulcer
- osteoporosis
- Cushing's syndrome

Antimalarials (chloroquine/hydroxychloroquine)

May be tried when NSAIDs have failed and before going on to steroids/gold/penicillamine:

Dosage: chloroquine 250 mg/day; hydroxychloroquine 200 mg twice daily
Side-effect: main one is retinal damage.

Immunotherapy

Indications:
- life-threatening extra-articular manifestations unresponsive to other treatment
- to allow a reduced dose of prednisolone (because of side-effects)

Dosage: azathioprine 1.25–2.5 mg/kg/day; cyclophosphamide 1–2 mg/kg/day
Side-effects: alopecia; bone marrow suppression; susceptibility to infection.

Indications for hospital referral in rheumatoid arthritis

- GP may want help with treatment.
- patient or family dissatisfied with progress.
- special problems – surgery needed, septic arthritis, difficulty in diagnosis.
- severe acute exacerbations – often settle better in hospital.

Indications for surgery in rheumatoid arthritis

- severe unremitting pain unresponsive to medical treatment.
- severe loss of joint function.
- severe joint instability.
- unacceptable loss of joint mobility.
- progressive joint destruction.

Types of surgery available

- synovectomy
- reconstruction of tendons
- arthroplasty
- arthrodesis

Acupuncture

This is claimed to relieve pain, stiffness and swelling in joints and muscles. Its place in the treatment of rheumatoid arthritis has yet to be established.

LETTER FROM CONSULTANT TO GP

Dear John,

Thank you for referring this retired greengrocer with a 3-month history of recurrent polyarthritis not responding satisfactorily to bed rest, aspirin, indomethacin and a short course of prednisolone.

I would think that the most likely diagnosis is rheumatoid arthritis, bearing in mind the pattern of joint involvement (elbows, wrists, knees, temporo-mandibular joint) and the positive rheumatoid factor test.

I have considered several other possible diagnoses but think them much less likely for the reasons stated:

Psoriatic arthropathy – *his skin rash is due to occupational dermatitis, his terminal phalangeal joints are not involved and his finger nails are normal.*
Gout – *the big toes are not involved and he has no tophi.*
Collagen disease – *the pains are not flitting, there is no systemic involvement (glands, heart, lungs, nerves, gastrointestinal tract or hypertension).*
Reiter's syndrome – *there is no conjunctivitis or urethritis.*
Systemic disease – *there is no abdominal pain or diarrhoea to suggest inflammatory bowel disease. There is no primary cause of amyloid and no other clinical manifestations (bowel, kidneys, hepatosplenomegaly). There is no evidence of sarcoidosis (respiratory glands, eyes or parotid). Occult malignancy always remains a possibility but would be a very rare cause of arthropathy.*

With respect to investigations, I would be interested in knowing the results of any joint X-rays you have had – otherwise I will arrange them. Apart from a collagen screen, I doubt if any other tests are really indicated.

As far as treatment is concerned, I think in the first instance I will arrange some physiotherapy and see how he gets on. Perhaps you might like to try him on antimalarials, such as hydroxychloroquine, and if this fails I think we will have to consider gold or penicillamine but it will be important to watch out for side-effects which can be serious.

He is not significantly disabled at present. If he gets to this stage, advice from an occupational therapist on a home visit would I am sure be helpful. A home nurse and a medical social worker may also be useful at an appropriate time.

Yours,

Gerald

- What do you think of the consultant's proposed actions?
- How do you interpret these to Mr and Mrs H?

OUTCOME

Five years later Mr H is still able to walk, but with difficulty, and to drive his car.

The chief site of the rheumatoid process are his knees. Both remain swollen with effusions and periarticular swelling in spite of removal of fluid and injection of steroids into the joints.

He is depressed and his morale is low. His wife also is depressed and tired.

The current medication is soluble aspirin up to 2.4 g and prednisone 10 mg daily.

PRACTICAL ISSUES

- What is the likely course over the next 5 years?
- What more can be done for his knees?
- How can help at home be organized in your district?
- What can be done for Mr and Mrs H's depression?
- How can the progression of rheumatoid disease be controlled?

SUBJECTS FOR DISCUSSION

- Epidemiology and natural history of rheumatoid arthritis (see Fry, J., Sandler, G. and Brooks, D. (1985) *Disease Data Book* (Lancaster: MTP).
- Effects on individual and family.
- Management policies – who should do what, where and how?
- Place of surgery in rheumatoid arthritis.
- Prevention and health promotion.

9 Chest Pain

MRS JANE S (AGED 59)

A medical receptionist in your practice who also runs a busy home with three teenage children. Her husband is manager of a supermarket store.

For 10 years she has experienced aching retrosternal chest on effort and emotional stress and worse in cold weather. Pain sometimes radiates to neck and jaw.

During this time she has also been awakened occasionally with chest pain. She has become more easily tired and breathless over the past 3 months.

Personal history

Happily married with a stable family.
Non-smoker and non-drinker. Walks whenever she can.
No previous history of ill health.

Family history

Father died at 41 from a sudden heart attack.
Mother is alive and well and is 79.
Three brothers – one aged 54 has had a stroke.

Examination

Height 5 foot 9 inches; weight 136 lbs.

Arcus senilis of both eyes.

Multiple xanthomata along extensor tendons of both hands and over both tendo achilles.

BP range: 150/86–170/95. Pulse regular 73.

No cardiac enlargement or abnormal heart sounds.

Chest sounds normal.

No oedema.

Investigations

ECG is normal

Chest X-ray – no cardiac enlargement

Serum cholesterol 14.41 mmol (normal is up to 6.7 mol)

Serum triglycerides 4.48 mmol (normal is less than 1.4 mmol)

Total HDL ratio is over 12 (normal average is 4.9)

- What is the presenting condition?
- What is likely cause?
- How do you interpret the results of the investigations?

MANAGEMENT

She has been on a low-fat diet for past 5 years and has kept her weight down. She is a most compliant patient.

Attempts to reduce her high cholesterol levels have been made with cholestyramine (and clofibrate). There was no reduction of cholesterol levels with these and they were unpleasant to take.

CHEST PAIN

- How would you treat her chest pains?
- What is your opinion of her BP levels?
- How would you manage her family?

THE GP's ASSESSMENT

Mrs Jane S is well known as a competent key member of the practice team who never fusses and is always calm and pleasant to everyone.

Clearly she has hypercholesterolaemia with angina over many years.

She has coped well but it is worrying that she has become breathless and fatigued over the past 3 months.

Recent ECG is normal and her heart is not enlarged.

Because of the personal relationship with Mrs S as a member of the practice staff a second opinion is considered necessary.

- How do you explain your action to Mrs S?
- What else would you discuss with her?

REFERRAL LETTER TO CONSULTANT

Dear Gerald,

Mrs Jane S (Aged 59)

Jane S is a valued member of our staff. An uncomplaining person who copes well with a large family and with part-time work in our practice.

For the past 3 months we have noticed that she is becoming breathless and fatigued – she admits to this reluctantly!

There is a long history (10 years) of angina on effort but occasionally also at rest and at night.

We know that she has hypercholesterolaemia and that her father died from 'a coronary' at 41 and probably he was also hypercholesterolaemic. A brother in his 50s has had a stroke. We have checked her children and their cholesterol levels are normal.

It is rather surprising, but gratifying, that her heart is not enlarged and ECG is normal.

She has been on a low-fat diet for years and we tried her on cholestyramine and clofibrate. Not only did they not reduce her cholesterol levels but she found them most unpleasant to take.

She has also been treated with glyceryl trinitrate for her angina, with relief and with beta-blockers, nifedepine and hydrochlorothiazide as a diuretic with no effects on her angina.

My problems are:
- *how else can we help her medically?*
- *how should we manage her as a member of our staff regarding her work?*

Yours

John

- What is your opinion of this referral letter?

CONSULTANT ASSESSMENT

The clinical problem is the management of a 59-year-old medical receptionist with a bad family history of cardiovascular disease and a 10-year history of angina who recently started to deteriorate with breathlessness and fatigue.

Management of angina

The aims of treatment are:

- to relieve symptoms
- to improve cardiac function

- to prevent complications:
    myocardial infarction
    cardiac arrhythmia
    sudden death
- to prolong life

Of these aims, modern treatment can effectively control symptoms and help myocardial function, but regrettably to date, convincing evidence that the development of a first myocardial infarction and/or sudden death can be prevented by either medical or surgical means has not been forthcoming. However, beta-blockers have been clearly shown to prevent a second infarction and coronary artery bypass surgery may be shown in the future to improve prognosis in multivessel coronary artery disease.

General treatment of angina

The main objectives are:

- STOP SMOKING;
- control hypertension;
- reduce blood cholesterol level;
- reduce obesity;
- treat anaemia;
- alter life-style.

Specific treatment of angina
Medical

The drugs which are available include:

- nitrates: *short-acting* to relieve or prevent an attack, e.g. glyceryl trinitrate, nitrolingual spray; *long-acting* for longer-term prophylaxis.
- beta-blockers.

- calcium-antagonists: especially useful where coronary spasm is suspected.

Surgical

The two types of surgery now in common use are:

- percutaneous coronary angioplasty – mainly used for single-vessel disease;
- coronary bypass surgery – for multivessel disease.

Management of hyperlipidaemia

The three major risk factors for coronary disease are:

- high blood cholesterol;
- cigarette smoking;
- hypertension.

Other risk factors include:

- family history;
- diabetes;
- obesity;
- contraceptive pill;
- 'soft' water;
- lack of exercise.

Hypercholesterolaemia

The evidence linking blood cholesterol levels and coronary disease is unequivocal. Regrettably, evidence that control of hypercholesterolaemia, except at the highest levels, produces significant benefits for patients remains unconvincing.

In the present state of knowledge, the indications for active treatment of hyperlipidaemia would include:

- a bad family history of *premature* coronary or other vascular disease (say under 50 years old);
- a young patient, say under 40;
- established ischaemic heart disease;
- very high cholesterol levels, especially if the LDL-cholesterol, the atherogenic fraction, is also high;
- other serious coronary risk factors are present – smoking, hypertension, diabetes;
- the presence of xanthoma, xanthelasma or premature arcus senilis.

The treatment of hyperlipidaemia is based on:

- a low cholesterol diet;
- the use of specific drugs:
    anion-exchange resins: cholestyramine, cholestipol;
    fibric acid drugs: clofibrate, bezafibrate, gemfibrozil;
    other drugs: nicotinic acid, probucol, Maxepa (conc fish oil), HMG co-reductase inhibitors: simvastatin

Analysis of GP's letter

History

Mrs S has had typical effort-induced angina for 10 years; this would suggest atherosclerotic coronary arteries. The nocturnal angina indicates the likelihood of associated coronary spasm.

The recent deterioration with breathlessness and fatigue raises the possibility of early left ventricular failure.

The premature death of her father at 41 from a heart attack may have resulted from hypercholesterolaemia and this could be familial. It also enhances the urgent need to achieve optimal control of Mrs S's angina as quickly as possible.

Examination findings

Arcus senilis in young patients, say under 40, suggests hyperlipidaemia and the possibility of premature arterial disease. At 59 however, I would not regard the arcus as of the same significance.

The xanthomata are more indicative of familial hypercholesterolaemia.

I would not regard the blood pressure as significantly increased (this would probably not be the view in the USA).

The absence of cardiac enlargement, gallop rhythm and pulmonary crepitations is encouraging in showing good left ventricular function.

Investigations

- *ECG*: the absence of left ventricular hypertrophy is a favourable prognostic factor.
- *Chest X-ray*: similarly, the absence of cardiac enlargement is favourable.
- *Blood lipids*: the cholesterol level is very high and would be consistent with familial hypercholesterolaemia. This diagnosis would be supported by a high LDL-cholesterol; triglycerides are either normal or mildly elevated in this condition, so that the triglyceride level of 4.8 mmol/l fits in with this diagnosis. Men affected by this condition show a 10-fold excess risk of developing coronary disease – as in Mrs S's father – but the risk in women is also substantially increased – as in Mrs S herself.

Management

Angina

Mrs S's angina has been treated with glyceryl trinitrate, beta-blockers and the calcium antagonist nifedipine. These three groups of drugs are the mainstay of medical treatment of angina but unfortunately Mrs S is not adequately controlled. Two other preparations which would be worth considering are longer-acting sorbide mononitrate and a transdermal nitrate such as a Transiderm-Nitro patch, which is particularly useful for nocturnal angina.

Breathlessness

The mild diuretic, hydrochlorothiazide, has been used but there is no indication as to whether the breathlessness has improved.

Hyperlipidaemia

Mrs S has failed to respond to a low-fat diet, cholestyramine and clofibrate. There are some other drugs available which would be worth considering, such as nicotinic acid, probucol, maxepa and simvastatin.

CONSULTANT'S LETTER TO THE GP

Dear John,

Thank you for referring this 59-year-old lady with long-standing angina and hypercholesterolaemia who is starting to deteriorate. I note also her bad family history.

As usual, I have gone into the history in some detail and I was concerned particularly by the recent exacerbation of her long-standing angina: whereas previously it had followed the typical pattern of precipitation by exertion or stress, it is now tending to occur at rest, especially in bed; this indicates that the angina is becoming 'unstable' which always raises the spectre of an impending infarction (20–25%) and therefore the need for more intensive treatment of the angina.

The other symptom which I thought significant and worrying was the recent breathlessness suggesting that she was developing early left ventricular failure: the recent fatigue could also be a manifestation of this

I examined her carefully and noted the arcus senilis and the xanthomata along the tendons due to the hypercholesterolaemia. I agree that there is no evidence of left ventricular failure at present – she was not dyspnoeic, there was no gallop rhythm and the lung bases were clear. The blood pressure was increased to 190/105 at the beginning of the examination falling to 170/100 at the end.

As far as treatment is concerned I think this should be considered under three headings – the angina, the left ventricular failure, and the lipidaemia.

She does require additional treatment for the angina and in the first instance I would like to confirm that she is on full dose of nifedipine, 20 mg t.d.s. I would also like to suggest a longer-acting nitrate preparation if this has not been tried already – either sorbide mononitrate or a transdermal stick-on patch such as Transiderm-Nitro (this might be especially useful for the nocturnal angina if she sticks it on when she goes to bed at night). If the angina remains a severe problem in spite of the additional treatment then we could always take her into hospital for a few days for more intensive treatment such as intravenous sorbide nitrate or heparin which I have often found of value in intractable angina. In the longer-term, if the angina remains disabling I think it would be worth considering Mrs S for coronary bypass surgery.

I note that you are treating the heart failure with a relatively mild thiazide diuretic; perhaps a more potent loop diuretic such as frusemide or bumetanide might be more effective. If the breathing does not improve adequately then a small dose of an angiotensin-converting enzyme inhibitor such as captopril, 12.5 mg b.d., or enalapril, 2.5 mg daily, would be worth a trial; the additional advantage of an ACE inhibitor is the beneficial effect on the blood pressure.

The last problem is the hypercholesterolaemia, which I note has not responded to a low-fat diet, cholestyramine and clofibrate. One additional specific suggestion I could make is to try a combination of cholestyramine and either nicotinic acid or probucol as both these combinations have been found to be more effective than cholestyramine alone in severe hypercholesterolaemia, and especially in the familial type which I think is likely in Mrs S.

Another alternative approach is to try the new HMG co-reductase inhibitor simvaststin (lovastatin in the USA) which has been found to be effective in resistant patients.

Finally, you ask about Mrs S continuing in the practice as your receptionist. If the angina and breathlessness respond satisfactorily to treatment and she wishes to continue working, then I would see no medical objection. I appreciate that there is a lot of stress involved in the work of a practice receptionist which could well exacerbate her angina and the only additional suggestion I would make to help the angina is to encourage Mrs S to use her trinitrin tablets as freely as possible to prevent the pain.

Please let me know if she doesn't settle down satisfactorily and I will then be happy to consider the next phase of her treatment.

Yours,

Gerald

OUTCOME

One year later Mrs S has been able to continue in the practice but working fewer hours.

Following the consultation it was insisted that she had a month's leave and rest.

She did not wish to take any more drugs apart from the glyceryl trinitrate tablets.

- What is the prognosis?

PRACTICAL ISSUES

- It is difficult to manage an inherited metabolic disorder for which there is no reliable or satisfactory treatment.
- It is often best to treat the individual patient rather than the disease.
- Prognosis is often better than may be expected from textbooks.
- An optimistic approach to patient care is justifiable even when the final outcome may be poor.

SUBJECTS FOR GROUP DISCUSSION

- What is the significance of hypercholesterolaemia in the community?
- How should it be picked up, managed and with what benefits?
- Problems related to care of one's own family and practice staff.

10 Funny Turns

PATRICK M (AGED 38) PART-TIME SECURITY GUARD

Always 'liked a drink'. Now increasingly getting involved in brawls – some very violent and not always associated with drunkenness.

Complains of headaches (diffuse)

Wife very worried by behaviour. She says she has noticed him having 'funny turns' – he looks dazed and seems not to notice her for periods up to a minute. She say's that his drinking mates complain of his bad temper.

He seems depressed and his alcohol intake is increasing.

Personal history

Married with four children. Marriage is under strain and children are afraid of him.

Came over from Ireland 19 years ago. Hasn't had a full time job for about two years, because of his unsatisfactory attendances and poor quality of work.

Serious car accident two years ago – thrown through front windscreen. Sustained skull fracture, dislocated right shoulder and multiple lacerations.

Drinks – six to ten pints (12–20 units) of beer a day, no spirits. Smokes – 20 cigarettes a day.

Examination

Height 6 foot 2 inches. Weight 13 stone 10 pounds.
Large scar on left forehead (from accident).
Complexion slightly florid.
No enlarged liver/no spider naevi.
No neurological deficit found.

- What other clinical stigmata of alcoholism would you look for?
- What neurological examination would you carry out?

Investigations

Hb 15.8 g/dl (normal M, 13.5–17.5 g/dl: F, 12.0–16.0 g/dl)
MCV 105% (normal 76–94 μ^3)
Gamma-GT 35 U/l (normal M, 9–50 U/l: F, 8–40 U/l)
SGPT 16 U/l (normal 8–20 U/l)
SGOT U/l (normal 8–20 U/l)
Bilirubin 5 μmol/l (normal 3–21 μmol/l)
Skull X-ray old fracture left temporal bone.

- Are there any other investigations you might think appropriate?
- Is the gamma-GT level always raised in cases of alcoholism?

MANAGEMENT SO FAR

Patrick agrees to come to the surgery with his wife (she has a black eye but explains that she fell down the stairs).

He admits to being depressed and to drinking too much. He denies marital or job worries as a cause. He says he is getting worried about his violence. Sometimes 'everything seems to go blank'. He says he has no knowledge of his funny turns his wife talks about, although he has noticed he keeps imagining he can smell oranges.

He eventually admits hitting his wife but says he does not know why he did it.

He is advised to cut down his drinking and is seen weekly in the surgery for support.

Three weeks later he is arrested and released on bail after seriously beating his next door neighbour.

The following week he is seen as an emergency at home after apparently having a grand mal seizure. He had been drinking that night.

- If he has an alcohol problem was this the best way to deal with him?
- Would you have treated his depression at this stage? If so, how?

THE GP'S ASSESSMENT

Patrick is drinking a lot, but there are no signs either on examination or after investigation of any liver damage.

He is certainly depressed.

He is getting what sound like absence attacks.

His problems seem to have begun around the time of his accident and appear to be getting worse.

REFERRAL LETTER TO CONSULTANT

Dear Gerald,

Patrick M (Aged 38)

Can you offer any help to this patient to prevent him from seriously injuring himself and/or someone else.

Patrick was an infrequent visitor to the practice until about two years ago when he was involved in a major road traffic accident which fractured his skull and dislocated his left shoulder.

He has always been a bit of a drinker, but recently he has been drinking heavily (six to ten pints (12–20 units)) despite being advised against it.

He admits to being depressed and has recently become quite aggressive often with no provocation. He has beaten his wife once to my knowledge and is now involved in a criminal assault charge.

His wife has noticed numerous 'funny turns' that sound like absence attacks. He almost certainly had a grand mal fit at home today.

My initial reaction was that his symptoms were all linked to his drinking. However his unprovoked aggression, absence attacks and history of a head injury make me wonder if there may in fact be some neurological cause – temporal lobe epilepsy crossed my mind. I wonder if you could have a look at him and give me your opinion as to the root cause. I would be extremely interested to see the result of an EEG.

Yours,

Martin Godfrey

- Should this referral be an emergency?

CONSULTANT'S ASSESSMENT

The clinical problem is a heavy-drinking 38-year-old security guard who had a serious head injury two years earlier and who has now become increasingly violent with the development of a grand mal fit.

The differential diagnosis of the violent behaviour and more significantly the epileptic fit in this patient should include:

- the effects of alcoholism;
- brain damage following the injury;
- the development of late-onset epilepsy;
- coincidental development of a brain tumour.

Alcoholism

Alcohol can damage the brain and produce several neuropsychiatric syndromes:

- *Korsakow's psychosis* – memory loss for recent events, confabulation.
- *Wernicke's encephalopathy* – difficulty in concentration; mental confusion; slowing of thought and speech; unsteadiness; focal neurological signs:
    diplopia
    nystagmus
    ophthalmoplegia
- *delirium tremens* – sudden withdrawal of alcohol.
- *dementia* – due to cerebral atrophy.

Head injury

Epilepsy may follow a serious head injury. The clues which suggest the likely development of post traumatic epilepsy are:

- long-lasting post-traumatic amnesia;
- depressed skull fracture with a dural tear;
- focal neurological signs;
- early epileptic fit (within the first week).

Late-onset epilepsy

The manifestations of temporal lobe epilepsy include:

- psychomotor seizures – characterized by abnormal behaviour patterns which may be pointless (e.g. picking at clothes, walking aimlessly), or highly skilled (e.g. driving a car, playing a musical instrument);
- various types of aura (hallucinations):
    unusual smell, taste or sound
    déjà vu
    alteration in size of objects
    formed sensory hallucinations
    feeling of acute anxiety or dread
- grand mal fits;

Abnormalities of behaviour are also more frequent in patients with temporal lobe epilepsy and may include attacks of explosive aggression.

Brain tumour

The sudden onset of a grand mal fit in a patient of 38 should always suggest the possibility of a brain tumour. The sites which can lead to a fit and are most frequently associated with impairment of mental function and alteration of behaviour are:

- corpus callosum
- frontal lobe
- right temporal lobe

Consultant's assessment of Dr Godfrey's findings
Alcoholism

Although Patrick is a heavy drinker he has so far not developed any significant liver disease based on the absence of any clinical findings of cirrhosis and the normal liver enzymes. However, the only definitive way of deciding whether there is any alcoholic hepatitis is by liver biopsy and this might be worth considering in Patrick's case.

There are other physical manifestations of alcoholism which should be sought in an alcoholic:

- *anaemia* – due to blood loss from the gastrointestinal tract and/or folic acid deficiency
- *peripheral neuropathy* – Dr Godfrey found no evidence of this on clinical examination
- *cardiomyopathy* – manifesting as cardiac arrhythmia (especially atrial fibrillation) and heart failure
- *cerebellar degeneration* – also excluded in Dr Godfrey's examination.

It would be helpful to know whether Patrick's attacks of violence on his wife and neighbours are related to his bouts of drinking, in which case this is the most likely cause.

Depression

Patrick is depressed but this could be due, at least in part, to the difficulty he has had in finding employment even though he does not readily admit this. Depression is also a frequent occurrence in alcoholism but is not a particular feature of temporal lobe epilepsy.

Alteration in consciousness

The patient's complaint of 'everything going blank' needs further clarification as it may well be a manifestation of temporal lobe epilepsy. The wife's description of 'funny turns' during which he looks 'dazed' and doesn't notice her for up to one minute would lend support to this diagnosis.

The hallucination of 'smelling oranges' is strongly suggestive of temporal lobe epilepsy.

Grand mal fit

The grand mal fit obviously requires further assessment. Fits are not a common manifestation of any of the types of brain damage due to alcoholism. It is important to decide whether the fit is caused by underlying brain damage resulting either from his previous head injury or from the coincidental development of a brain tumour.

Headache

The 'diffuse headache' needs clarification, particularly with reference to the possibility of raised intracranial pressure, the features of which are:

- throbbing
- site: occipital – infratentorial tumour; frontal – supratentorial tumour
- worse at night and on walking
- worse on straining, e.g. coughing, sneezing, bending
- associated nausea and vomiting
- blurring of vision

An alternative diagnosis which also needs to be considered is 'tension' headache which presents with:

- character: pressure, tight band, heavy weight
- often at vertex but may occur at any site
- lasts hours or days
- worse at times of stress
- other symptoms of anxiety

Investigations done by the GP

Mean corpuscular volume

The increased mean corpuscular volume suggests folic acid deficiency in spite of the normal haemoglobin; this can occur with alcoholism.

Liver function tests

The normal results exclude serious liver involvement as a result of the alcoholism.

Skull X-ray

This confirms the old fracture. There are no signs of a brain tumour such as:

- a displaced pineal gland
- calcification, e.g. meningioma, astrocytoma
- enlarged vascular channels, e.g. angioma
- bony erosions, e.g. neoplastic metastases, myeloma
- increased bone density – meningioma
- eroded sella turcica – pituitary tumour
- eroded petrous temporal – acoustic neuroma

However, a skull X-ray has a poor predictive value for brain tumour.

CONSULTANT'S LETTER TO THE GP

Dear Martin,

Thank you for referring this 38-year-old patient who is a heavy drinker. I note that you are concerned about his violent behaviour, his 'funny turns' and a recent grand mal fit. You are wondering whether these symptoms might all be related either to a serious head injury two years earlier possibly causing temporal lobe epilepsy or to the alcoholism.

In the first instance, I have gone into the history in some detail with Mr M and his wife and think that the 'funny turns' are indeed due to epilepsy arising in the temporal lobe. The smell of oranges is, I am sure, a temporal lobe aura, particularly as this often precedes the onset of the 'funny turns'. I have also gone into this complaint in some detail; what he apparently means by 'funny turns' and 'blankness' is the surroundings suddenly seeming far away and unreal – a typical partial seizure of temporal lobe origin. The grand mal fit is also probably triggered by a temporal lobe focus spreading to the cerebrum generally. The important question is to decide whether the temporal lobe epilepsy is primary or secondary to an organic lesion of the temporal lobe, and, if secondary, can it be related to brain damage caused by the road traffic accident or is there the coincidental development of a brain tumour?

The diffuse headache is likely to be a tension headache as he describes a feeling of heaviness over the whole of his head which usually lasts for hours at a time, and sometimes for days. I agree also with your findings that there are no abnormal neurological signs and in particular no evidence of raised intracranial pressure. The answer to the question of an organic temporal lobe lesion is going to depend on a CT brain scan and I will get this done as soon as possible and let you have the result. An EEG may be of value in showing a focal dysrhythmia in the temporal lobe but if it is negative it will not be of any diagnostic help at all: with these reservations, however, there would be no harm in doing one and I will arrange this also.

As far as treatment of the temporal lobe epilepsy is concerned this will obviously depend on whether an organic lesion is found in the temporal lobe; if so, then a neurosurgical opinion will be required. If the CT scan is negative, then it would be worth treating the epilepsy with an anticonvulsant such as carbamazepine: if the 'funny turns' are satisfactorily controlled with the drug it would be interesting to see whether this altered his aggression also.

I have tried to assess the problem of the alcoholism as well. I examined him for any stigmata of cirrhosis and, like you, found none; nor could I find any evidence of cardiomyopathy, peripheral neuropathy or cerebellar dysfunction. I have not gone into his neuropsychiatric state in any great detail but he does have a poor memory and poor concentration – then who hasn't these days? – I certainly do! More specifically, I found no evidence of mental confusion or confabulation: his speech is not impaired and there were no focal neurological signs in the cranial nerves to suggest a Wernicke encephalopathy. I am checking on his blood folate levels in view of the macrocytosis, and if low, then folic acid supplements would be desirable. I think we can defer the question of the liver biopsy for the present as there is no indication so far of any clinical liver problem.

I have explained to Mr and Mrs M that he needs further investigation and treatment of the fit, and I have indicated the possibility that the bouts of aggression may be part of the same problem. I have also pointed out that he is drinking far too much, and although it has not produced any serious complications so far, it is likely to cause severe damage to his liver, heart and brain some time in the future. It may be of help for him to see a psychiatrist and get some further advice and, if I may, I will leave the decision about this to you and Mr M as no doubt you will want to discuss this with him in more detail and at more length, I think he has been a bit shaken by what I said about the long-term effects of his drinking and I hope this will provide the necessary motivation to want to do something about it.

Yours,

Gerald

OUTCOME

CT scan showed the presence of a high-density lesion in the right temporal lobe about 2 cm in diameter.

EEG confirmed temporal lobe epilepsy which a characteristic discharge consisting of sharp spikes and slow waves in the right temporal lobe region.

A phone call to the local neurosurgical unit obtained a bed that afternoon.

Mr M was asked to attend the surgery urgently and when seen was told bluntly that he has a brain tumour. He was obviously very shaken by this news and began weeping. He declined the offer of an ambulance to take him up to the hospital saying his wife would drive him there.

That night, at about midnight Mrs M asked for a home visit. Mr M had barricaded himself in the front room and was obviously very drunk. He became aggressive when told that the doctor was in the house saying 'he will never be taken into the hospital'. Despite various remonstrations he refused to come out. His wife said there was an amount of whisky in the room. After about an hour his mood altered and he sounded tearful. He threatened to kill himself.

The police were called and Mr M was eventually escorted quietly to the hospital. Surgery three days later allowed the removal of a small meningioma.

Post-operatively he made a good recovery although unfortunately he had developed an upper quadrantic hemianopia, worse on the right than the left side.

He did not resume his drinking following the enforced abstinence brought about in hospital. His funny turns ceased.

- Why has the hemianopia developed?
- What other focal neurological lesions often develop with lesions in the temporal lobe?
- What typical radiological finding is often seen in skull X-rays of patients with a meningioma?

PRACTICAL ISSUES

- It is very often a mistake to jump to the most obvious conclusions in a case, even when it seems to be staring you in the face. It would

have been very easy to consign all Mr M's symptoms to alcohol; much valuable time could have been lost in preventing permanent neurological damage if such a conclusion had been made without considering the differential diagnosis.
- A case such as this is very damaging to the family. They will often need as much support as the patient.
- There are many schools of thought about the best way of telling patients they have cancer. In this case Mr M was told coldly that he had a tumour, with no explanation of the likely outcome or treatment that he would receive. Many people regard the development of cancer as a death sentence, thus every effort should be made to offer them as much support as is possible in the circumstances.

SUBJECTS FOR GROUP DISCUSSION

- Alcoholism and its treatment in general practice.
- Signs and symptoms of cerebral tumours.
- Who tells a patient he has cancer and how should it be done?
- Dealing with violent patients.

11 Dizziness

JAMES M (AGED 76)

A retired foundry worker who used to work on blast furnaces. He lives with his wife in a flat.

Mr M is well known to the practice for over 30 years. Mrs M is the dominant partner.

For over 10 years 'Jimmy' has come intermittently for 'dizzy turns'. More recently he has fallen in the street. The attacks are becoming more frequent and appear to be brought on by sudden movements.

His hearing has been progressively worse for many years and he wears a hearing aid, which he cannot manage very well and he is bothered by high-pitched noises in both ears.

Personal history

James M is an uncomplaining man who is pushed into doing things by his wife (he has confided that he is glad that he can 'turn a deaf ear' to her sometimes).

He worked in the local foundry from the age of 14 to 65. His hobby is pigeon racing and he has 20 pigeons in his back garden. A heavy smoker, he has a constant productive cough. Has 'a few pints of beer' each week.

Past history

Apart from his dizzy attacks, he has suffered from bouts of bronchitis and pneumonia.

Examination

Slight and wizened. Old for his age.
Chest is emphysematous and the peak flow rate is 210 l/min
CVS: small heart
BP: 165/105 (sitting); 160/100 (standing)
Pulse rate: 76 regular
Neck: stiffness in all directions; carotid arteries feel arteriosclerotic
Ears: drums look normal but with some wax in meati
CNS: no nystagmus; fundi normal; negative Romberg's test; gait normal.

- What are the possible causes of Mr M's symptoms?
- What investigations would you order and why?
- How would you manage Mr and Mrs M and why?

MANAGEMENT

You endeavour to explain to Mr and Mrs M that the likely cause of James's symptoms are damage to his ear nerves from his past work in the foundry and also some hardening of the arteries of his neck.

You offer to get some tests carried out, such as X-rays of his neck, hearing test and blood tests, but Mrs M wants Jimmy 'to see a specialist'!

- How do you respond to Mrs M's request?
- Why do you think she wants a referral?

THE GP'S ASSESSMENT

James M is a hen-pecked man who is dominated by his wife, she has become fed up by the recurrent bouts of dizziness.

The cause of his symptoms is most likely to be a combination of auditory-labyrinthine damage from occupational acoustic trauma, plus increasing cerebrovascular insufficiency.

There is no effective treatment for these symptoms.

This is a classical situation for a 'therapeutic referral', for no other reason than to seek support from a specialist colleague for a non-curable situation.

- What is your opinion of such an assessment?
- List main reasons for referral to a specialist.
- What is the range of referral rates among GPs? What is your own referral rate – if you don't know, how would you measure it?

REFERRAL LETTER TO CONSULTANT

Dear Gerald,

Mr James M (Aged 76)

James M is suffering from recurring bouts of dizziness, hearing loss and tinnitus. His wife is more bothered by them than he. The relationship between them is less than warm.

My own assessment is that his symptoms are consequences of old acoustic nerve trauma from his work at the local foundry and from cerebrovascular insufficiency.

I have suggested to them that there is nothing specific to be done apart from taking care not to move too quickly.

I have referred him really at the insistence of his wife who demanded to 'see a specialist'! I hope that you will agree with my assessment and reinforce my message to them.

Yours,

John

> • What is your opinion of this referral letter?

CONSULTANT'S ASSESSMENT

The clinical problem is the management of an elderly patient with a long-standing history of deafness, tinnitus and dizziness which is getting worse and now leading to frequent falls.

The first thing to consider when a patient complains of dizziness is what is actually meant by the complaint. The possible meanings are:

- true vertigo
- an impending faint
- light-headedness
- loss of balance.

Having established the nature of the complaint, the various causes should then be considered.

Vertigo

- vertebro-basilar insufficiency
- Meniere's disease
- middle-ear disease
- vestibular neuronitis
- benign positional vertigo
- acoustic neuroma
- cerebello-pontine angle tumour
- drugs – salicylates, phenytoin, quinine, streptomycin/gentamycin

Faint

- cardiac: Stokes–Adams attack, myocardial infarction, aortic/pulmonary stenosis
- vasomotor – simple faint (vasovagal attack), prolonged standing
- cough/micturition syncope
- hypoglycaemia

Light-headed

- cerebrovascular insufficiency
- anaemia
- anxiety/hyperventilation
- drugs, especially peripheral vasodilators for hypertension

There is one more differential diagnosis that needs to be considered in the light of Mr M's falls and that is the causes of sudden falls in an elderly patient:

- Stokes–Adams attack
- drop attacks due to vertebro-basilar ischaemia
- severe postural hypotension
- epilepsy (akinetic type)

CONSULTANT'S ANALYSIS OF THE GP's LETTER

History

Attacks of dizziness

The sudden falls, precipitated by movement, could well be 'drop attacks' associated with vertebrobasilar insufficiency. To confirm the diagnosis, it would be necessary to establish that there was no previous warning, rapid recovery and no residual symptoms. It would also be important to exclude an attack of vertigo which might be accompanied by tinnitus and nausea and which could be due to Meniere's disease.

Deafness

The progressive deafness and the 41 years in the iron foundry is very suggestive of noise-induced hearing loss. This is particularly prone to occur with prolonged exposure to drop-forging and the use of percussive tools. It is due to damage to the Organ of Corti in the inner ear with gradual deterioration of the sound-sensitive hair cells and degeneration of the auditory nerves.

Confirmation of the diagnosis can be obtained from the audiogram, which typically shows bilateral hearing loss of 40 dB or more at frequencies over 2 kHz.

Tinnitus

Tinnitus is common in noise-induced labyrinthine damage and often predates the patient's own perception of his deafness.

Heavy smoking and productive cough

This obviously suggests the likelihood of chronic bronchitis, and the clinical examination shows evidence of emphysema also. The importance of this in relation to dizziness is that a prolonged bout of coughing may produce syncope (cough epilepsy). As Mr M's dizziness and falls have presumably not been preceded by prolonged coughing, 'cough epilepsy' is not relevant.

Examination findings
Ear findings

Blockage of the external auditory meati with wax can cause deafness and may also sometimes lead to vertigo, so this should be kept in mind as a possible contributory factor in the recent exacerbation of his symptoms.

Neck stiffness

This is no doubt due to his cervical spondylosis which may be causing vertebrobasilar insufficiency.

The carotid arteries are arteriosclerotic which will aggravate the development of cerebrovascular insufficiency.

Another useful diagnosis sign of carotid stenosis is the presence of a murmur over the carotid artery in the neck.

Neurological signs

The negative neurological examination, particularly the cranial nerves, would exclude an acoustic neuroma, and the normal fundi would also tend to exclude any other type of brain tumour in the cerebello-pontine angle.

It is not clear whether Mr M's hearing was tested in the course of the examination: apart from confirming the deafness, the Weber and Rinne tests might help in showing whether the deafness was due to middle ear or inner ear disease.

	Weber	*Rinne*
Middle ear disease	affected side	bone > air
Inner ear disease	normal side	air > bone (both reduced)

Nystagmus is sometimes present in chronic labyrinthine disorders but it is not present in Mr M. It is unusual to find any focal neurological signs in brain-stem insufficiency in between attacks.

CONSULTANT'S LETTER TO THE GP

Dear John,

Many thanks for referring this elderly patient with deafness, dizzy turns and some recent falls.

I have gone into the history in some detail. The dizzy turns consist of a feeling of light-headedness or faintness which I agree is very suggestive of vertebro-basilar insufficiency. An additional relevant symptom is that he admits that the dizziness is worse with sudden head movements, like looking to the side or even more so if he looks upwards suddenly; this suggests that he has cervical spondylosis also which is causing compression of the vertebral arteries on neck movement and is playing an important part in his dizziness.

As far as the falls are concerned, he told me he has no warning beforehand but just falls suddenly with no loss of consciousness and is then able to get up almost immediately and feels quite all right afterwards. These are typical 'drop attacks' due to vertebro-basilar insufficiency.

On examination, I confirmed the limitations of such neck movements indicating cervical spondylosis and was able to hear a systolic murmur over both carotid arteries in the neck indicating carotid stenosis.

I found that his deafness was more in the left ear; the Weber test was referred to the right ear and air conduction was better than bone conduction in both ears (Rinne test) but both were reduced compared with my own hearing – this indicates clearly that he has labyrinthine disease on both sides which fits in with a diagnosis of noise-induced hearing loss.

I could not find any abnormality in the examination of the nervous system so that I do not think we need to consider a more sinister cause for the dizziness, like an acoustic neuroma or other types of intracranial tumour, and I do not think, therefore, that he needs any detailed neurological investigations such as a CT scan.

In the cardiovascular system, the relevant points are that there is no evidence of any likely source of emboli which might cause transient ischaemic attacks – in particular, he is not fibrillating and he does not have valvular heart disease. He does have severe arteriosclerosis with thickened tortuous radial and brachial arteries, absent foot pulses and fundal arteriolar changes; this obviously supports the diagnosis of cerebrovascular insuffi-

ciency. His blood pressure is increased, as you pointed out, my readings being 170/105 both in the lying and standing position.

As far as investigations are concerned, we could do an X-ray of his cervical spine which will confirm the spondylosis but we know this already, from our clinical assessment, though I suppose it may also show carotid calcification which would be of prognostic value. Brain scans (isotope or CT) are likely to be negative, so I doubt if they are worth doing. There is nothing to suggest Stokes-Adams attacks so there is little point in 24 hour ambulatory ECG monitoring. The only diagnostic test which would be helpful is audiometry which may well show the typical picture of noise-induced deafness, and I shall arrange this and let you have the result when it is to hand.

As far as management is concerned, as you mentioned in your letter, there is very little to be done for his deafness, though it might be worth trying a hearing aid which is occasionally of some value.

With respect to his dizziness, I would suggest that he try a plastic collar if he can be persuaded to wear this for as much of the day as possible. It might also be worth starting him on a 75 mg dose of aspirin to prevent platelet-induced thrombosis in the atherosclerotic carotid arteries in the neck in the hope of averting a cerebral embolus.

Finally, although he has a mild degree of hypertension I would be disinclined to treat this as it may well aggravate the dizziness due to the cerebrovascular insufficiency.

Yours,

Gerald

OUTCOME

Mr M's dizziness settled considerably after being given the cervical collar, although in the opinion of the ENT surgeon who subsequently saw him, Meniere's syndrome was the most likely cause.

In view of the diminution of symptoms no other therapy was thought necessary.

One year later Mr M was still having the occasional attack of dizziness, but rarely came to the surgery complaining about them.

Both he and Mrs M blame the condition on his past work.

- Why does Meniere's syndrome occur?

PRACTICAL ISSUES

- The appearance of a patient complaining of dizziness often makes the GP's heart sink since the diagnosis is difficult and the treatment often unsatisfactory. It is well to remember, however, that 'dizziness' can mean many things (true vertigo, an impending faint, and so on) thus it is important that the true identity of the symptom is ascertained.
- Tinnitus can be an extremely debilitating condition and should not be ignored, although little can be done to help.
- In this case the dominating spouse got things done, but often an over-vocal husband or wife can blur the picture of what is going on. Make sure you get as much information as possible from the patients themselves.

SUBJECTS FOR GROUP DISCUSSION

- Can you construct a useful protocol for examining dizzy patients?
- What drugs are commonly used in the treatment of dizziness, how do they work and what side-effects do they have?
- How do you deal with ear wax?

12 Back Pain

MRS JENNY P (AGED 61)

Mrs P is an ex-nurse living with her husband, who is unemployed, and a teenage daughter.

She is a frequent attender with a fat folder. Her main complaints over the past 15 years have been tiredness and backache.

The marriage is an unhappy one. Mr P has been out of work for 3 years, since the local printing press shut down. He is a heavy drinker and smoker and keeps her short of money. At times he has hit her.

The reasons for her present consultation are more severe backache since she strained it on lifting 10 days ago. She can hardly move now and the pain is waking her at night.

She is a non-smoker and does not drink. Bowels and micturition are normal. No weight loss.

Past history

Her depression has been treated by anti-depressants at various times and also she has been prescribed analgesics and non-steroidal anti-inflammatory drugs for her backache. She has had periods of physiotherapy without lasting relief. Records show that she has had referrals to gynaecologists for heavy menses and menopausal symptoms; to rheumatologists for backache; and to psychiatrists for depression. None of these referrals helped her very much.

Examination

She looks unwell and is obviously in considerable pain in lower back. She looks pale and is breathless.

She stands in a bent posture and there is tenderness over lower lumbar region. Movements are restricted because of pain. Attempts at straight leg raising are difficult because of pain in back. Leg reflexes are normal.

There are no abnormalities in chest, breasts, cardiovascular system (BP 150/85) and abdomen.

- What is your assessment of Mrs P's case so far?
- List possible diagnoses.
- What would you do next?

Investigations

Blood report (summary): Hb 6.9 g/dl (normal 12–16 g/dl); MCV: 82.4 fl (normal 76–94 fl); ESR 98 mm/hour (normal 5–15 mm/hour).

X-ray report of lumbo-sacral region: narrowing of L4/5 and L5–S1 spaces; there is collapse of L4.

- What is the most likely diagnosis?
- What other investigations would you order?

MANAGEMENT

By the time the reports are received Mrs P is unable to come to the office and she is visited at home.

BACK PAIN

There is no change in her condition. Her husband is surly and aggressive and demands that something is done quickly so that she can look after him.

This is a situation that requires a domiciliary consultation.

> - What is a domiciliary consultation (DC) and how can it be arranged?
> - What are usual indications for a DC?

THE GP's ASSESSMENT

Mrs P has suffered for many years from depression and backache.

Home and marital situation is bad with a non-caring aggressive husband.

Present situation is new with low backache severe enough to make her housebound.

Blood test shows severe anaemia and very high ESR.

X-ray reports collapse of L4.

She is a very ill lady and the most likely diagnosis is myelomatosis.

CONTACT WITH CONSULTANT

GP phones consultant (specialist) to arrange for a DC and following points are made:

- Mrs P has severe low backache with severe anaemia and high ESR, and myelomatosis is a possibility.
- she cannot attend hospital for consultation.
- the family situation is fraught and a DC may reduce tension all round prior to admission.

DC is arranged and GP and consultant meet and attend together. Mr P and daughter are present.

CONSULTANT'S ASSESSMENT

The clinical problem is a lady of 61 with a long-standing back problem and now presents with worsening back pain, severe anaemia, a high ESR and a collapsed lumbar vertebra on X-ray. The main problems which need elucidating are:

- the cause of the severe back pain
- why she has become so anaemic
- whether the high ESR is due to malignancy
- whether the collapsed vertebra is also due to malignancy

Back pain

The causes of back pain are legion: it is helpful to consider them under acute and chronic.

Acute

- prolapsed intervertebral disc
- vertebral collapse due to osteoporosis
- acute infection – pyogenic, tuberculosis
- neoplasms – carcinomatous metastases, myeloma, reticulosis

Chronic

- chronic disc prolapse
- osteo-arthrosis
- ankylosing spondylitis
- tuberculosis
- congenital, e.g. spondylolisthesis
- psychogenic

Tiredness

Tiredness, weakness, lassitude and lack of energy are very common complaints and often very difficult to elucidate, especially as these symptoms are frequently present in the absence of organic disease. However, it is prudent to consider all the possible organic causes in a particular patient before dismissing the complaint as 'functional'. Among the causes which need to be considered are:

- anaemia
- infections – viral, e.g. glandular fever, hepatitis, tuberculosis, infective endocarditis, other rarities, e.g. brucellosis
- endocrine – myxoedema, Addison's disease, hypopituitarism
- metabolic – uraemia, diabetes, cirrhosis
- drugs – tranquillisers, hypnotics
- malignancy
- severe cardio-respiratory disease

High ESR

This should always cause considerable concern in a middle-aged or elderly patient as, in the vast majority of cases, it indicates serious organic disease. Causes which need to be considered include:

- carcinomatosis
- myelomatosis
- giant cell arteritis, e.g. temporal arteritis
- polymyalgia rheumatica
- collagen disease, e.g. SLE, scleroderma, polyarteritis nodosa
- infections especially pulmonary, urinary tract
- rarities, e.g. Wegener's granulomatosis, left atrial myxoma

Anaemia

The causes of anaemia are many and the diagnosis depends on its type and mode of onset. Among the causes which need to be considered are:

Iron deficiency

- inadequate intake of iron (especially old people)
- excessive iron loss: gastrointestinal – piles, peptic ulcer, drugs (e.g. NSAIDs), varices (cirrhosis); uterine – menorrhagia, fibroids

Macrocytic

- vitamin B12 deficiency: pernicious anaemia, Crohn's disease

Haemolytic

- intrinsic defects: congenital spherocytosis, thalassaemia, sickle-cell anaemia
- extrinsic factors: auto-immune; drugs – methyl dopa, quinine; cold haemoglobinuria; hyperspenism (any cause); mismatched transfusion; rhesus incompatibility

Normocytic (of uncertain origin)

- chronic disease – rheumatoid arthritis, chronic infection, liver disease, uraemia
- malignancy

BACK PAIN

Causes of collapsed lumbar vertebra

In the absence of appropriate trauma, the causes which need to be considered include:

- osteoporosis
- hyperparathyroidism
- myeloma
- secondary carcinoma – bronchus, breast, stomach, kidney, colon, thyroid, prostate

CONSULTANT'S ANALYSIS OF THE CLINICAL POINTS MENTIONED BY THE GP IN HIS 'PHONE CALL

History

Depression

Mrs P does have a lot of domestic stress with her husband who is a drinker and violent on occasions, a good basis for anxiety, depression and psychogenic fatigue: there is also a past history of post-natal depression severe enough to require ECT treatment. There is a strong temptation, therefore, for the doctor to attribute her symptoms to her mental state and the home problem – this initial response must be resisted! It is the wiser course to regard Mrs P as an organic case until proved otherwise. When likely organic causes have been excluded then the possibility of a recurrence of a depressive illness can be considered, and in this case she would be expected to have other manifestations of depression such as:

- insomnia
- early waking
- loss of interest
- lack of concentration
- loss of libido
- anorexia

- constipation
- loss of weight

Tiredness

As the tiredness has been present for 15 years it is unlikely to be due to any serious organic cause. Long-standing iron-deficiency anaemia is a possible cause, especially in view of the current severe anaemia found by the GP: if this is the case, she might have some helpful signs on examination, like koilonychia or glossitis. Alternatively, it could have a psychological origin. Unless there has been a sudden acute exacerbation of the tiredness it is unlikely to be related to malignancy in view of its prolonged duration.

Back pain

Although Mrs P has a long history of back pain, it would appear from the letter that the pain has never been as severe before. This raises the possibility that she has developed a new cause of back pain and taken with the X-ray findings of a collapsed 4th lumbar vertebra, it is highly likely that such a lesion is malignant.

Examination findings
Pallor

This indicates anaemia. There is no mention of either koilonychia (chronic iron deficiency) or an atrophic tongue (pernicious anaemia): both conditions are possible causes of anaemia in a lady of this age. The other condition which needs to be kept in mind is malignancy.

BACK PAIN

Spinal findings

The tenderness over the lower lumbar region is very suspicious of a lesion in the bodies of these vertebrae – most likely carcinomatous or myelomatous deposits – but will require further tests to be sure.

The normal leg reflexes would be against root involvement, especially from a disc lesion.

Investigations

Blood count

This shows severe anaemia but in the absence of additional information on red cell parameters and the blood film appearance, it is not possible to suggest a definite cause at this stage, though marrow infiltration would obviously be a likely cause.

ESR

The very high ESR is the most important abnormality and is clearly likely to be due to serious organic disease, with neoplasm high on the list of possible causes.

X-ray spine

The collapse of L4 raises the possibility of carcinoma or myeloma. In the absence of any comment on osteoporosis in the rest of the spine, this is very unlikely to be the cause.

The narrowing of L4/L5 and L5/S1 disc spaces indicate prolapsed intervertebral discs in the past.

CONSULTANT'S LETTER TO THE GP

Dear John,

Thank you for asking me to come with you to do a domiciliary consultation on this 61-year-old lady with a long-standing back problem which has become much more acute recently. I noted also her long-standing tiredness, the severe anaemia, the high ESR and, most significantly, the collapsed lumbar vertebra. As I promised after our discussion at Mrs P's home, I am now putting my views down on paper for the patient's records.

On going into the history, it appears that the recent back pain is quite different to the chronic backache. Although the site is similar, the chronic backache has been dull, related to movement of the spine and often radiating to the lower limbs – this is obviously a lumbago/sciatica type of syndrome probably due to a chronic disc problem with superadded degenerative changes in the spine. The current severe pain started fairly suddenly about 2 weeks ago – she attributes it to lifting a heavy shopping bag, but this may be coincidental rather than causal. The pain is much more severe than her previous back pain, doesn't radiate to the legs and is present at rest, especially at night in bed: this sound very suspicious to me of a focal lesion in the vertebral body, most commonly malignant.

Support for this diagnosis is provided by the loss of about a stone in weight since the onset of the pain and a marked loss of her appetite. The fatigue is unlikely to be relevant to a possible diagnosis of malignancy because it has been present for so many years. She thinks that the tiredness may be getting worse recently, but this could well be due to the severe anaemia.

I can add little to your findings. She is obviously anaemic but she does not have koilonychia or atrophy of the tongue thus excluding chronic iron deficiency and pernicious anaemia as likely causes. I have confirmed the local tenderness over L5 but have not found any other evidence of a metastatic condition such as enlarged glands or hepatomegaly, and I could not feel a spleen to suggest reticulosis.

The high ESR and the collapsed lumbar vertebra are obviously highly suggestive of malignancy. She needs to be admitted urgently for investigation: chest x-ray to exclude primary or secondary neoplasm, x-ray of lumbar spine for malignant deposits including myeloma, urine examination for Bence-Jones protein, serum electrophoresis for myeloma and bone marrow examination for carcinoma, myeloma or reticulosis.

I have discussed the problem with Mrs P and suggested that she may have 'inflammation' in the spine without mentioning the probability of malignancy. I have a feeling though, that she is aware of and fearful of this diagnosis. However, she did not openly raise the matter and I felt at the present time it was unjustifiable to alarm her unduly, at least until we were sure of the diagnosis. She has agreed to come into hospital as soon as we can arrange a bed.

Yours,

Gerald

OUTCOME

X-ray of Mrs P's lumbar spine showed punched out lytic lesions in the body of L4 with collapse.

The chest X-ray didn't show any evidence of bronchial carcinoma.

Serum electrophoresis showed a tall narrow M spike thus confirming the diagnosis of myeloma. Further confirmation of this diagnosis was obtained from the bone marrow examination which showed extensive infiltration with plasma cells.

Bence-Jones protein was found in the urine.

Mrs M was informed of the diagnosis and was given radiotherapy to the spine which was very effective in relieving her back pain, for which she was very grateful. She was subsequently started on melphalan and prednisolone and sent home to continue treatment.

PRACTICAL ISSUES

- This was a confusing case, but because of the severity of the condition it is not one that could be ignored for long.
- A knowledge of the patient's family was obviously very useful in this case.
- A single symptom (such as backache) is usually caused by a single condition, but on occasion this rule can lead to confusion.
- The diagnosis and treatment of back pain, in all its guises, is one of the greatest burdens a GP must bear.

SUBJECTS FOR GROUP DISCUSSION

- Discuss the pathophysiology involved in multiple myeloma.
- How does the GP become involved when a patient is receiving chemotherapy?
- What special problems occur in families that have children very late in life?

Index

abdominal disease, pain caused by, 51
abdominal pain (in the 'never well'
  patient), 47, 51–2, 53–4
  causes, 51–2
  diagnosis, 52
  character, 53
  site, 52
absence attacks, 103, 104
acoustic nerve trauma, 117, *see also*
  auditory nerve degeneration
acupuncture in rheumatoid arthritis,
  85
aggressive behaviour, *see* violent behaviour
airways disease, chronic obstructive,
  see obstructive airways disease
alcoholism, 35–45
  diagnosis, 38–9
  management, 40–2
    difficulties in, 44
  manifestations, clinical and physical, 39, 40–2, 105, 107, 111
  in patient with 'funny turns' and
    previous head injury, 101, 103,
    104, 105, 107
  practical issues, 44, 102–3
ampicillin in chronic bronchitis, 33
anaemia
  alcohol abuse-related, 39, 41, 107
  in the back pain patient, 130, 132
  causes, 39, 130

iron deficiency, 130, 132
  pallor indicating, 132
angina, 95, 96–7, 97, 98
  complications, 93
  management, 92–4, 96–7, 98, 99
angiotensin converting enzyme
  (ACE) inhibitor therapy
  in heart failure, 98
  in hypertension, 18, 20
antibiotics
  in chronic bronchitis, 30, 32–3, 33
  hepatotoxic, 5
anticonvulsant drugs, 110
antihypertensive drugs
  compliance with, 17
  fluid retention caused by, 72
  hepatotoxic, 5
anti-inflammatory drugs, hepatotoxic,
  5
antimalarial drugs in rheumatoid arthritis therapy, 84
arcus senilis suggesting hyperlipidaemia/hypercholesterolaemia,
  96, 98
arthritis, rheumatoid, 77–88
  investigations and diagnosis, 80, 81,
    86
  management, 81–5
  practical issues, 87
asthma
  bronchial, diagnosis, 29

INDEX

chronic bronchitis with, 31–2
  late onset, 26, 31
  management, 30
atenolol, 1, 2, 3
auditory nerve degeneration, 120, *see also* acoustic nerve trauma
aura (hallucinations), 106, 108, 110

back pain, 125–36
  acute/recent, 128, 134
  causes, 128
  chronic, 128, 134
  practical issues, 136
balance, loss of (= sudden falls), causes, 119
blood pressure
  high, *see* hypertension
  mildly elevated, 8
  in swollen leg patient, 68, 75
blood tests, *see also specific tests*
  in back pain patient, 126, 127, 133
  in chest pain patient, 96
  in 'funny turns' patient, 109
  in recurrent polyarthritis, 80–1
bowel, muscle spasm in, pain due to, 55
brain
  alcohol-related damage, 42, 107
  tumour, in patient with 'funny turns', 106–7, 112, 113
breathlessness, 25–34
  in chest pain patient, 91, 97, 99
    management, 97, 99
  in swollen leg patient, 70–1
bronchitis
  chronic
    asthma with, 31–2
    diagnosis, 28, 31, 120
    practical issues in, 34
    treatment, 29–30
  wheezy, diagnosis, 29
bronchodilators, 30, 32
  aerosol, 30
  in asthma, 30

cancer/malignancy, *see also* tumours
  in back pain patient, 132, 133, 134, 135
  fear/dread, 55, 113
    in the 'never well' patient, 55
  informing patient of, 113
captopril, in heart failure, 98
carbamazepine, 110
cardiomyopathy, alcohol-related, 42, 107
cerebellar degeneration, alcohol-related, 42, 107
cerebrovascular insufficiency, 117, 121, 122–3
cervical spondylosis, *see* spondylosis, cervical
chest pain, 89–100
  practical issues, 99–100
chloroquine in rheumatoid arthritis therapy, 84
cholesterol levels
  high, *see* hypercholesterolaemia
  tests, in chest pain patient, 96
cholestyramine, 90, 97
  nicotinic acid or probucol combined with, 98–9
cirrhosis, alcoholic, 39, 42
  treatment, 40–1
clofibrate, 90, 97
colitis, ulcerative, X-ray radiography in, 80
collagen disease, diagnosis, 81, 86
consciousness, alteration in, 107–8
coronary disease, risk factors, 94
corpuscular volume, mean, in patient with 'funny turns', 109
cough, productive, smoking and, in patient with dizziness, 120
Crohn's disease, X-ray radiography in, 80
cromoglycate in asthma, 31

deafness (hearing loss), 117, 118, 120, 122

INDEX

delirium tremens, 105
dementia, alcohol-related, 105
depression
    in back pain patient, 131–2
    in 'funny turns' patients, 101, 103, 104, 107
    manifestations, 131–2
dihydroergotamine mesylate, 57–8, 60
diuretic therapy
    in heart failure, 98
    in hypertension, 19–20
dizziness, 115–24
    causes, 118–19
    practical issues, 124
doctors, specialist and family, communications between, 23
drop attacks, 119, 122
drugs, *see also specific drugs*
    in angina therapy, 93–4, 96–7
    antibiotic, *see* antibiotics
    anticonvulsant, 110
    antihypertensive, *see* antihypertensive drugs
    anti-inflammatory, 5
    fluid retention caused by, 72
    hepatotoxic, 5
    in hyperlipidaemia therapy, 95
    psychotropic, 5
    in rheumatoid arthritis therapy, 81, 83–4
dyspepsia, persistent, 35–45

ear examination in patient with dizziness, 120
electrocardiography in chest pain patient, 96
electroencephalography in patient with 'funny turns', 110, 112
emphysema, 120
enalapril
    in heart failure, 98
    in hypertension, 20, 20–1
encephalopathy, Wernicke's, alcohol-induced, 41, 105

endocrine disorders, hypertension associated with, 17
epilepsy
    diagnosis, 110
        differential, 105–6
    late-onset, 106
    manifestations, 106
    seizures and fits in, 103, 104, 105, 106, 108, 110
    temporal lobe, 104, 106, 107–8, 107, 110
    treatment, 110
ergot preparations, 61–2
    toxicity/side-effects, 62
ergotamine, 57–8, 60, 65
erythrocyte sedimentation rate in the back pain patient, 129, 133

faint, impending, causes, 119
falls, sudden, causes, 119, 122
'fat-folder' syndrome, 49, 52
fatigue (tiredness) in the back pain patient, 129, 132
fits and seizures, 103, 104, 105, 106, 108, 110
fluid retention caused by drugs, 72
flu-like illness, jaundice preceded by, 5
'funny turns', patient with, 101–13

gold drugs in rheumatoid arthritis therapy, 83
gout, diagnosis, 80, 86
grand mal fits/seizures, 103, 104, 105, 106, 108, 110
gynaecological disease, abdominal pain caused by, 51, 52

haemolytic anaemia, 130
haemolytic features in jaundice, 4
hallucinations, 106, 108, 110
head injury, 'funny turns' in patient with previous, 101, 105–6, *see also* skull

INDEX

headaches, 57–66
  causes, 60–1, 108, 110
    diagnostic features, 63, 110
    diffuse, 108, 110
    in patient with 'funny turns', 108
  practical issues, 66
  tension, *see* tension headache
health promotion relating to hypertension, 22
hearing loss (deafness), 117, 118, 120, 122
heart failure
  in chest pain-presenting patient, 97, 98
    management, 98
  hypertension causing, 72
hepatitis, infective, 2, 9
  diagnosis, 9
hepatitis A infection, 11
hepatocellular features in jaundice, 4
hepatotoxic drugs, 5
HLA typing, diagnosis via, 81
home nurses for the rheumatoid arthritis patient, 82
hospital referral in rheumatoid arthritis, 85
hydroxychloroquine in rheumatoid arthritis therapy, 84
hypercholesterolaemia (high cholesterol levels), 91, 91–2, 94, 98–9
  management, 90, 94, 98–9
hyperlipidaemia
  arcus senilis suggesting, 96, 98
  management, 94–5, 97
  indications for, 95
hypertension (high blood pressure)
  causes, 7, 10, 13–23, 72
  clinical significance, 15–16
  headaches associated with, 63
  jaundice and, 3, 4, 7–8, 10
  practical issues in, 21–2
  primary/essential, 7, 18
  resistant, 13–23
    problems of, 16–17
  risk factors associated with, 16, 21
  secondary, 7, 17
  target organ damage in, 7–8, 16, 72
  treatment for, 8, 17, 18, 19–20, 72, *see also* antihypertensive drugs

immunotherapy in rheumatoid arthritis, 84
infection in chronic bronchitis, 30, 32–3
inhalers (in breathlessness management), problems with, 32
intracranial pressure, raised, diagnostic features, 63
iron deficiency anaemia, 130, 132

jaundice, 1–11
  causes, 4
  clinical features, 4
joint pains, multiple, 77–88, *see also* arthritis; polyarthritis
  practical issues, 87

kidney (renal) disease, hypertension associated with, 17, 18
Korsakow's psychosis, alcohol-related, 41, 105

legs, swollen, 67–75
  causes, 70
  practical issues, 75
light-headedness, causes, 119
limbs, lower, *see* legs
lipids, blood, in chest pain patient, 96
liver function tests
  in 'funny turns' patient, 109
  in jaundice, 6
lumbar vertebrae, collapse, causes, 131
lumbo-sacral region, X-rays of, in back pain patient, 126, 127, 128, 133, 135
lymphatic oedema in swollen leg patient, 71

INDEX

macrocytic anaemia, 130
malignancy, *see* cancer
maxillary sinusitis, headaches related to, 64
Maxolon, 62
mean corpuscular volume in patient with 'funny turns', 109
Meniere's disease, 119
meningioma in patient with 'funny turns', 112
methyl xanthines in asthma, 31
migraine
   diagnostic features, 63
   headaches untypical of, 59, 60
   prophylaxis, 65
   treatment, 61
Migraleve, 62
Migravess, 62
Migril, 62
mini-peak flow meters, 32, 33
muscle spasm in bowel, pain due to, 55

neck stiffness in patient with dizziness, 121, 122
neurological disease/neuropathy
   abdominal pain caused by, 51
   alcohol-induced, 41
   dizziness associated with, 121
neuropathy, peripheral, alcohol abuse-related, 107
'never well' patient, 47–55
nicotinic acid combined with cholestyramine, 98–9
nitrates in angina therapy, 93–4
nurses, home, for the rheumatoid arthritis patient, 82
nystagmus, 121

obesity
   hypertension and, 22
   swollen legs patient with, 67, 74
obstruction, local, swollen legs caused by, 70

obstructive airways disease
   chronic, 26
   diagnosis, 28
obstructive features in jaundice, 4
occupational therapy in rheumatoid arthritis, 82
oedema, leg, in swollen leg patient, 71–2
organs, target, in hypertension, 7–8, 16, 72

pain, *see specific site of pain*
pallor in the back pain patient, indications, 132
pancreatitis, alcohol-induced, 41
peak flow meters, mini-, 32, 33
penicillamine in rheumatoid arthritis therapy, 83
physicians, specialist and family, communications between, 23
physiotherapy in rheumatoid arthritis, 82
pizotifen, 65
placebos, headache patient response to injections of, 65
polyarthritis, acute and recurrent, 77–88
   cause, diagnosis, 79–81
probucol combined with cholestyramine, 98–9
psoriasis/psoriatic arthropathy, diagnosis, 86
   investigations in the, 80, 81
psychiatric/psychological symptoms/manifestations
   of alcoholism, 39, 41, 105
   in the 'never well' patient, 49, 53
psychiatric/psychological treatment in alcoholism, 40, 43
psychogenic causes
   of abdominal pain, 51, 53
   of headache, *see* tension headache
psychomotor seizures, 106
psychosis, Korsakow's, alcohol--

related, 41, 105
psychotropic drugs, hepatotoxicity, 5
pyelography, intravenous (IVP), 18

radiography, X-ray, *see* X-rays
Reiter's syndrome, diagnosis of, 86
  investigations in the, 80, 81
renal disease, hypertension associated with, 17, 18
rheumatoid arthritis, *see* arthritis, rheumatoid
rheumatoid factor, positive, significance, 79–80
Rinne's test, 121, 122

sarcoidosis, blood tests in, 80–1
seizures and fits, 103, 104, 105, 106, 108, 110
sinusitis, headaches relating to, 59, 64
skull
  fracture, in patient with 'funny turns', previous, 101, 105–6
  X-ray, in patient with 'funny turns', 109
smoking
  alcohol abuse and, 43
  and productive cough, in patient with dizziness, 120
social services for the rheumatoid arthritis patient, 82
spasm, muscle, in bowel, pain due to, 55
specialists and family doctors, communications between, 23
spine in back pain patient, 133
  X-rays of, 126, 127, 128, 133, 135
spondylosis, cervical
  dizziness associated with, 121, 122
  headaches associated with, 63, 64–5
steroids
  in asthma therapy, 31
  in rheumatoid arthritis therapy, 83–4
surgery
  for angina, 94
  for rheumatoid arthritis, 85
swollen legs, *see* legs
systemic disease, recurrent arthritis caused by, 79
  diagnosis, 86

temporal lobe, organic lesions, 110
temporal lobe epilepsy, 104, 106, 107–8, 107, 110
tension, in mind and muscle, muscle spasm in bowel caused by, 55
tension headache, 60–1, 110
  diagnosis, 63, 64, 108, 110
thrombosis, venous/deep vein, in swollen leg patient, 69, 71–2, 73
tinnitus, 117, 118, 120, 124
tiredness in the back pain patient, 129, 132
tobacco smoking, *see* smoking
triglyceride levels in chest pain patient, 96
tumour, brain, in patient with 'funny turns', 106–7, 112, 113, *see also* cancer

ulcerative colitis, X-ray radiography in, 80

vasodilators for hypertension, 72
venous oedema in swollen leg patient, 71
venous thrombosis in swollen leg patient, 69, 71-2, 73
ventricular failure, left
  in chest pain-presenting patient, 97, 98
  management, 98
  hypertension causing, 72
vertebrae, lumbar, collapse, causes, 131
vertebrobasilar insufficiency, 121, 122
vertigo, causes, 118, 120
violent behaviour in patient with

INDEX

'funny turns', 103, 104, 105
  differential diagnosis, 105–6

Weber's test, 121, 122
weight, over-, *see* obesity
Wernicke's encephalopathy, alcohol-induced, 41, 105

xanthomata, 96, 98

X-rays
  chest, in chest pain patient, 96
  of joints, in recurrent polyarthritis, 80
  skull, in patient with 'funny turns', 109
  spinal, in back pain patient, 126, 127, 128, 133, 135